ASSESS | REBUILD | CONNECT

Assess

Rebuild

Connect

CREATING
A NEW LIFE
BEYOND
ADDICTION

ADAMS RECOVERY CENTER

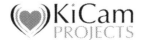

Cover and book design by Mark Sullivan

ISBN 978-0-9991581-2-8 (paperback)
ISBN 978-0-9991581-3-5 (e-book)
Library of Congress Control Number: 2018938217

Printed in the United States of America

Published by KiCam Projects
www.KiCamProjects.com

CONTENTS

If you have picked up this book, we hope you are working toward maintaining your sobriety or helping a loved one maintain his or her sobriety. We believe that when it comes to addiction, knowledge is power, and our hope is that through this book, as well as the first two books in this series, we can create understanding about why people affected by addiction might act the way they do. We also hope to start a real conversation about the problems facing us nationwide related to addiction.

As you read through these pages, we believe they'll help you start a conversation about addiction closer to home—with your loved ones, peers, significant other, and even in your community in general. Addiction is a life-or-death issue. Our intent is not to scare you, but rather to remind you that you can make a huge difference in your own life, in the lives of those close to you, and in the lives of your coworkers and neighbors who need support.

That all starts with understanding, which is why we wrote this book to address a number of concepts relevant to people in early recovery. We'll explore how individuals in the post-treatment stage can cope with the many firsts they experience in their new lives of sobriety, as well as how they can rebuild trust, navigate family dynamics and communication, learn to live with integrity, find new passions unrelated to using, and manage medical issues in ways that are healthful both physically and emotionally.

Often, we encounter the misconception that once someone goes through a treatment program, he or she will be "fixed." But in fact, sobriety is a long-term work in progress. Our hope for this book is that it will introduce you to concepts and topics you might not have considered and inspire you to explore some of the thought processes that occur in addiction. We hope you'll be both encouraged and challenged to think and act in ways that foster successful, lifelong sobriety for yourself and those you love.

Our Program

ARC is an agency dedicated to change. We are a separate-gender drug and alcohol treatment program. We offer residential, intensive outpatient, and individual counseling services. Our program is a modified Therapeutic Community running the Hazelden clinical curriculum. We use the latest evidence-based practices and incorporate cognitive behavioral therapy, rational-emotive behavior therapy, and behavior therapy to maximize client gains in the program.

Our inpatient program is designed for an approximate one-hundred-eighty-day stay. Our staff includes drug and alcohol counselors, mental health counselors, nurses, and medical doctors.

ARC embraced the Therapeutic Community model due to its renowned success worldwide. The Therapeutic Community is recognized and endorsed by the United States federal government. Within the T.C., clients (called "sisters," "brothers," or "the family" collectively) come out of their denial and into acceptance regarding their substance abuse. Clients expose their thinking errors and learn how to look at people, places, and things differently. The T.C. is a residential hierarchy in which every resident has a job (for example, cleaning the kitchen, taking out the trash, inspecting the dorms, etc.). Clients engage in several hours of group therapy per day, in addition to individual counseling and case management.

We do not believe that one size fits all when it comes to treatment, and we do not believe we can simply hand clients answers. Instead, we help them find their own.

When a client has made sufficient evident clinical and personal progress at ARC, the client graduates and is referred for aftercare. We make sure our graduates feel comfortable and confident in themselves and in their aftercare plans.

Many of our clients go on to live successful lives free of substances, and we love hearing from these clients and celebrating their continued progress.

Our Staff

The staff at ARC comprises individuals who are certified or licensed in various disciplines. All clinical staff hold, at the minimum, certifications as chemical dependency counselors (CDCA) in the state of Ohio. Most staff are licensed as chemical dependency counselors (LCDC, Level 2 and Level 3), and others hold Licensed Independent Chemical Dependency Counselor (LICDC) designations. Multiple staff members hold the LICDC-CS, which is the clinical supervisory endorsement—the highest form of chemical dependency licensure in Ohio.

We have a Licensed Professional Counselor (LPC) who is certified in Ohio, and our medical coordinator is a Registered Nurse who holds a CDCA.

We come from various counseling backgrounds, from a variety of schools of thought. We draw from cognitive behavioral therapy, behavior therapy, rational-emotive behavior therapy, reality therapy, choice therapy, existential/gestalt therapy, and other diverse therapeutic orientations, which allows multiple techniques and interventions to be used.

Several members of our staff contributed to this book in order to provide multiple perspectives.

We are happy you picked up this book and hope it serves you in whatever ways you need. Though obviously our work focuses on treating drug and alcohol addiction, the topics discussed in these pages apply to virtually anyone and can help you or those you care about reach whatever goals you're striving for!

CHAPTER ONE

A Quick Overview

Just as you and your loved ones have been on a journey in sobriety, we at Adams Recovery Center have been on a journey of helping others achieve that goal. This book, the third in a series, represents just one step in our efforts to reach people whose lives are affected by addiction. In the two previous books, we touched on many topics related to addiction. Perhaps you read them a long time ago and need a refresher on some of the more significant points. Maybe you skipped the first two, finding this one more relevant to your current needs. Whatever the case, we'll revisit some crucial concepts to make sure we are all on the same page before you continue reading. So, let's get started.

ADDICTION: WHAT IT IS AND WHAT IT ISN'T

Perhaps your thoughts are: *Why are you defining addiction in a book about addiction?* If you're holding this book, you have a pretty clear understanding of addiction, right? Well, maybe. It's startling how many different definitions of "addiction" there are, just like there are many different definitions of "sobriety." If we are going to talk with you for an entire book, it's probably a good idea to let you know how we view addiction.

We tend to accept the standard definition that addiction is a physical and mental dependence on something—in this case, a substance—which is used regardless of the consequences it brings. You rely on the substance. Feel like you can't live without it. You *need* it. That leads us to determining whether the substance use is a problem.

In *Accept, Reflect, Commit*, we state that one question is enough to determine whether substance use is a problem: Is your use, in any way, having a negative impact on any aspect of your life?

We go on to discuss what can be done if the answer to this question is "yes," and we make suggestions for what steps to take in order to address the problem. Since you're reading this book, our hope is that you've gone through that process and are at least somewhat settled into a sober life. If this is the case, we are *so* happy for you. You've taken a huge step. Let's offer a gentle reminder, though: Addiction is truly a life-long process. It's not something that can be "cured" or forgotten once the substance is out of your system. We assume you know this already, but even those with years of sobriety under their belt sometimes need a reminder—and that's okay!

It's completely reasonable to want to put behind you something that caused so much destruction. At the same time, forgetting or neglecting things that are crucial to our health and wellness simply because they are painful to think about is irrational. Does a person with diabetes cease taking insulin and following an appropriate diet because it is too upsetting to acknowledge he has diabetes? We would hope not. It's the same thing with addiction. It is healthy to acknowledge the parts of ourselves, both physical and mental, that need constant maintenance. Everyone has their stuff. It's part of the human experience.

We encourage our clients (and *you*) to actively embrace this part of you. Living in shame and hiding away your past will only allow it to continue to haunt you. Addiction is not a defect. It is not a moral weakness, a punishment, or a characteristic of someone who is lesser. Society wants to pigeonhole addiction and those who struggle with it into certain categories, and media often presents it as something to be feared. Don't get us wrong—addiction itself *is* scary, but believing that the reality of your life is to be feared will only continue to let it rule you.

Maintenance in Sobriety

Addiction is one of those things that needs constant maintenance. As humans, it is healthy that we view ourselves as constant works-in-progress rather than already perfect beings. If you think your only issue in life is your addiction and, otherwise, you are flawless, then we are *super* concerned. Okay, so you might not think you're flawless, but have you ever thought that if you took the substance out of the equation, life would be pretty great? That your issues wouldn't really be issues? That's common. What people tend to forget is that addiction doesn't come out of nowhere, and it often develops in reaction to not utilizing healthy coping skills to handle issues—whether they be a major event or daily stressors.

If you have any length of sobriety under your belt, you're well aware that your other problems did not go away once the substance was gone. In fact, you may have begun to notice other problems you didn't even know existed! That's typical of the recovery experience. In fact, our previous two books focus primarily on these issues and how to navigate them. One thing we also make clear is that some things can be dealt with once and solved for good. Others, not so much. It might take weeks, months, years—a lifetime, even!—of regular processing and work on these things. Some things, such as stress management, are daily practices rather than one-time-solves-all. This is where maintenance comes in.

One visual we often use with the clients is thinking of our mental well-being (and, subsequently, sobriety) as a car. Obviously, owning a car is not as simple as buying it and driving it around forever until it someday dies. If only it were that easy! Unfortunately, owning a car requires so much regular maintenance: change the oil, make sure the fluids are at appropriate levels, clean the engine, change the tires, replace the brakes, take it through the car wash, vacuum it every once in a while—we could go on and on. It appears humans are often more willing to do these things for their cars than they are to care for themselves. Just like cars, we need constant care and maintenance, too.

If you've been to a treatment program, you (hopefully) spent plenty of time learning about and implementing various self-care and stress-management techniques. You may have even built up a pretty solid routine that you are still following now. Unfortunately, what happens for many, is that they allow "life" to take over and stop prioritizing these routines and practices that keep them healthy. You stop exercising as much. You go to fewer meetings. You haven't touched your journal in weeks. Your diet begins to include a lot more cheese. Slowly but surely, these things that helped you get well go by the wayside, and that is the perfect time for our old habits and unhealthy coping skills to return. This is often when people relapse.

As we previously stated, even those who have been sober for years sometimes need a reminder that constant self-care and assessment of self are needed to maintain sobriety. It is a lifelong process that will require trial and error and revaluation of needs and priorities. New life situations will arise, new relationships will develop, and new responsibilities will demand your attention. In the end, the priority *needs* to be your well-being and your sobriety. If those things no longer matter to you, it can be a slippery slope back to destructive mindsets and habits. Luckily for you, this book is full of advice and insights on how to navigate obstacles that might arise for you in early sobriety.

Continuing to Trust the Process

Hopefully, we've made it pretty clear so far that life in

sobriety will not always be perfect and easy. If we haven't, let's emphasize it now: *Life in sobriety will not be perfect and easy!*

A sober life will have many challenges and obstacles to overcome. The solutions to these problems will not always be apparent, and sometimes it will feel easier to just give up. This is when it is most important to continue trusting the process. In *Accept, Reflect, Commit*, we discuss what it means to "trust the process" and explain that, by doing so, we are essentially accepting life on life's terms rather than trying to force things into the mold we believe they should be in. To trust the process means to know and accept that if we consistently strive to make healthy decisions and move forward, life will happen the way it is meant to happen. We recognize that we have only a small amount of control over what goes on in the world, and that things will not always go our way. Trusting the process means trusting that life is worth living despite its negative moments. Those negative moments are simply part of the process and meant to serve as lessons.

Are you possibly groaning over how unrealistic this sounds? It's okay. In fact, many clients groan when we encourage them to trust the process. *Defining* trusting the process is a lot easier than, well, *actually* trusting the process. But that doesn't mean it's not a mindset worth pursuing. If you're currently sober, we are going to guess that you've had to challenge your perceptions of control in some way. Being addicted to something allows it to control you—your mood, your body, your priorities, your life. You know this; you've lived this. On the flip side, though, you engaged in your own controlling behaviors while in active addiction. Your primary focus was on obtaining your substance, and you controlled those around you and your environment in order to continue using. And, hey, we aren't judging here! We are just acknowledging what comes with addiction and what it can cause people to do.

When entering into sobriety, people often struggle with relinquishing control. It's difficult to put an end to these behaviors and adopt a new way of living. This is going to be difficult for anyone, let alone someone who has spent possibly decades living a lifestyle that supports addiction. What we tend to see happen, though, is that people accept the lack of control while in treatment but then begin to reintroduce these controlling behaviors when they are back in the "real world." In this book, we've made sure to address some situations that often re-awaken the control monster in people: regaining trust in loved ones, establishing routines and working toward goals, experiencing firsts in recovery, etc. These are all situations in which it will be crucial to trust the process and recognize that things will work out as they should. It is often during these challenging moments that we grow more fully into who we are meant to be and when we are given the opportunity to become better people.

Maybe you were hoping your mother would trust you with driving her car again after you'd been sober for a few months. However, it's been almost a year and she still won't even consider handing you the keys. Or, maybe you anticipated being able to juggle two jobs at once and now find yourself completely overwhelmed. Perhaps you believe it's time to get back out into the dating world, but you go on two dates and don't really feel that "spark" you expected to feel. Though stressful, these are all common situations that require trust in something greater than ourselves. We are not going to tell you what that thing needs to be. We simply refer to it as "the process."

By experiencing these things, you are able to learn and grow and allow yourself to further develop as an individual. Trying to force others to cater to your comfort level or trying to dominate a situation to generate a certain result may only make things worse and hinder progress on your goals. Constantly arguing with Mom over the car might cause her to tighten her grip on the keys; continuing to work two jobs despite the exhaustion it brings might cause you to further ignore your self-care and slip back into bad habits; settling for a relationship that does not actually interest you could lead to unnecessary drama and pain.

In order to trust the process, it's important to continue challenging your perceptions. Rather than having tunnel vision on the issue, try to take a step back, take in a deep (deeper, really) breath, and look at the entire picture. Ask yourself how you can learn from it, how you can cope with discomfort in a healthy way, and—be honest—how much will this "it's not going my way" situation matter a year from now? Keep these things in mind as you continue reading, and think about how you can apply trusting the process to the new challenges that await you. It'll all work out—we promise.

Realistic Expectations

If we are going to encourage you to trust the process, it only makes sense for us to briefly discuss those expectations you have. You know the ones—how you envision life and your future now that you're sober. It's natural to begin considering what all you can have and accomplish now that you are no longer living for your substance. And in many ways, that's awesome! You might be considering your ability to do things you never considered before, or you feel excitement over regaining things you thought were lost forever. These thoughts and plans are great motivators and can help you continue to take positive steps forward. On the other hand, if not kept in check, expectations can do more harm than good.

In our first book, *Addiction, Recovery, Change*, we discuss what it means to set realistic expectations, in addition to issues to keep in mind when navigating early sobriety. One thing we address is boredom and how this can be an issue people don't anticipate. A lifestyle of addiction brings a lot of intensity in both emotion and experience. Transitioning into a "normal life" is sometimes harder than people expect. There is no longer a daily struggle toward obtaining and using the substance, no more lies and manipulation, no more "crazy" experiences while in using environments. Now, it's all about a nine-to-five job, playing with your kids, and watching your favorite TV show. Oh. That's…normal. And not too exciting. (Now, stay with us here. *We* do not think this is boring, but we'll get there in a second.)

It's important to acknowledge that instead of striving toward balance and adjusting to the demands of daily living, people in early recovery might seek other ways to provide that high and distract themselves. This can come in many forms, whether it be developing unhealthy habits (for example, gambling) or turning to old friends. Returning to old, unhealthy relationships and habits out of boredom is one of the most dangerous things a person can do, and it often leads to relapse.

Readjusting to normal, daily life may take time—and that's okay! It might be a healthy expectation to set for yourself. Many times, people don't take this into account and then wonder what is wrong with them when they don't feel automatically fulfilled by their new life. Or, perhaps things are not moving at a pace they expected, and they wonder if they're ever going to accomplish their goals. Nothing is wrong with you! This is perfectly healthy. Here is where trusting the process comes back into play, too. By living each day the best you can, and challenging boredom in a healthy way, you're taking steps closer to fully embracing this new way of life. Often, boredom stems primarily from someone not feeling like he or she has a purpose or a drive in life—no greater, larger goal. If this applies to you, that's *normal.* Questioning purpose and drive in life is a very human thing to experience, and something everyone struggles with at some point, addict or not.

This is where the fun part comes in. Now that you're sober, you have *so* many opportunities out there! We don't just mean jobs either. We mean hobbies, experiences, people to meet, movies to watch, music to hear—the list goes on. By truly living without the cloud of your addiction hanging over your head, you're able to be fully present in those moments and note their impact. It is through our daily experiences, both boring and exciting, that we begin to learn more about ourselves and where our passions lie. It's really difficult to consider passion when we are catering to addiction. Without addiction, there are so many avenues that are now open to you. Later in this book, we talk more about passion and what that could look like in early recovery.

ARE YOU READY FOR THIS?

Here is our encouragement for you: Get excited about this time in your life! Embrace it. Love it. You're stepping into new territory, a place you've never been before. Sure, maybe you've had times of sobriety in the past, but that was the past. This is now. This is where your new life begins—and it can continue if you allow it. We've made it clear (maybe painfully so) that there will be struggle. It won't always be easy, and you will face challenges, possibly on a daily basis.

All of this can feel terrifying, and people in early recovery often ponder whether they are truly ready to do this sobriety thing. Do they really have what it takes? Are they actually able to move forward?

Yes. The answer is yes. Life can change as soon as you want it to and are willing to embrace it—all of it, the good and the bad. No one needs a natural set of skills or a certain personality type to live a sober life. It can happen for anyone at any time. Don't let the pressures of the outside world, the negative opinions of your family, the fear of having responsibilities, the uncertainty of the future—we could go on and on—hold you back. There is so much support available if you're willing to accept it, and you do not have to go through this alone. We encourage you to seek out those willing to help and support you. If you don't believe anyone out there exists, then we suggest stepping into a meeting room, a church, a community center—anywhere people with common interests gather—and see whom you can find.

In the meantime, though, you're holding this book right now, and it has tons of information in it that we believe will be helpful to bear in mind as you're on this journey. Take a breath, settle in, and enjoy the ride.

• • • JESSE'S STORY • • •

Jesse entered treatment after using meth heavily for five years. At first, he was skeptical of what treatment could do for him, but over time, he began to make positive changes and made significant progress toward his goals. Jesse found that incorporating daily exercise into his routine, plus nightly journaling, greatly helped his stress levels. When he graduated, Jesse was excited to enter into a sober-living facility and begin his new life.

Things went well for Jesse at first—he liked his roommate, he got a job, he was regularly attending meetings, and he maintained his daily exercise and journaling. Jesse's job began early in the morning and was located next to a convenience store. Every day, Jesse would stop into the store to pick up an energy drink to have before work. Soon, Jesse found himself stopping into the convenience store on his breaks to get another energy drink, and he would pick one up on his way home. Jesse was soon consuming up to four energy drinks a day, even on days he did not work. He began to notice he did not have as much spending money after his bills were paid, and he found himself feeling irritable more frequently. Jesse's roommate expressed concern over his fluctuating mood and noted that he hadn't seen Jesse work out or journal in a few weeks. Jesse initially rejected this concern, stating that he was fine and that he was just too busy with meetings and work to do those things.

During a session with his counselor, Jesse began to process his frequent irritability and stress. After the session, Jesse walked home and became even more irritated. *Why did he have to do so much to function? Why couldn't he just be a "normal" person? The energy drinks aren't that much of an issue—they aren't meth!*

When Jesse woke up the next morning, he felt exhausted, these things heavy on his mind. Jesse decided to reach out to some friends and met them for lunch. Jesse's friends reassured him that he is a "normal" person for needing to take time for himself and continue this exercise and journaling routine. Another friend also suggested he decrease the number of energy drinks he was consuming, preferably down to zero. Even though he was frustrated, Jesse chose to listen to the advice of his peers. That night, he worked out with his roommate and took five minutes to journal about his day. The next day, he drank only two energy drinks. A month later, Jesse was back to his routine and felt more at ease and less irritated. Jesse also stopped drinking the energy drinks and allowed himself only one small cup of coffee in the morning on his way to work.

Jesse continued to experience occasional irritation, and had some days where he did not exercise or journal, but overall, he trusted the process and continued to strive toward balance in his life.

For Reflection

- How do you feel about trusting the process? What does that mean to you, and how does it challenge you?

_____

_____

_____

_____

_____

_____

_____

_____

_____

- What are some factors in life that you've learned to control? What are some issues you've come to understand are out of your control?

_____

_____

_____

_____

_____

_____

_____

_____

- What are your expectations for life in sobriety?

_____

_____

_____

_____

_____

_____

_____

_____

- How do you define for yourself what it means to live a "normal life"?

  _____

  _____

  _____

  _____

  _____

  _____

  _____

  _____

- When you think about a new life beyond addiction, what excites you, and what causes you some anxiety?

  _____

  _____

  _____

  _____

  _____

  _____

  _____

  _____

CHAPTER TWO

Rebuilding Trust

One of the many challenges people face in long-term sobriety is understanding whom and how to trust. Typically, individuals in recovery *want* to trust others but struggle with the confidence to do so because of past broken trust and promises. What we hope to accomplish in this chapter is to help you find the right kind of trust.

To acquaint ourselves with the word itself, let's start with one of Merriam-Webster's definitions of trust, which is "one in which confidence is placed."

When you think about active addiction, in whom did you place confidence? Many times, it probably was people who weren't doing the right thing. You might have trusted the drug dealer to get the drugs you needed, or maybe it was the friend who could "hook you up with the good stuff." Why do you think you did this? What made you trust them?

It probably had something to do with past experience or knowledge of those people. They might have given you drugs before, or perhaps other people had told you they were good for whatever you were looking for.

Take some time to examine the roots of your trust issues. Was there a lack of trust in your family when you were growing up? Have people you trusted in the past let you down consistently? Or have you spent time in prisons or jails, where no one can be trusted? As you navigate this chapter, explore what is at the core of your trust problem, and identify what material here applies to your personal situation.

One goal of this book is to enable you to begin to trust your family, peers, and anyone else who is doing the next right thing.

Trusting Others

So, where do you go from here? Let's start with thinking of people you want to trust. Who are the people who have been there for you from day one? This could be family members, friends from school, friends from your recovery network, or members of a religious/spiritual group. At the end of this chapter, we'll make a list in writing.

What makes you want to trust them? Is it that they are non-judgmental? Do they see the world from the same viewpoint as you? Are they caring individuals? Do they maintain sobriety?

The "why" really matters here. Many times, in sobriety circles, you will hear that the "why" isn't important, but with trust, understanding the "why" helps identify and clarify your basic issues with trust in general.

Why do you want to share something personal with someone? Is it because you need to share something important for your own sobriety, or is it to help the other person?

Is there something eating at you that could lead to relapse? Do you just need moral support?

Recognizing why you want to share things with a particular individual will help you recognize the bigger purpose of trust. Take Alcoholics Anonymous, for example. It has become such a key piece of sobriety for many people because attendees trust that nothing will be repeated outside the support group. They believe that other members of the group can relate to their problems and will keep their stories confidential, without judgment.

There is no doubt that various anonymous groups work for many people. That said, sobriety doesn't require that level of all-or-nothing thinking when it comes to trust. In sobriety—as with life in general—it's not necessary to give everyone complete trust about every detail of your life. Some issues might be best confided in a friend. Others might be suited for a family member. Still other topics might lend themselves to being shared with a professional.

For example, let's say you are an intravenous drug user and have contracted HIV from sharing a needle that was infected. Naturally, such a discovery feels overwhelming. Not only do you have to figure out what you are going to do medically, but you have to face your fear of dying from the disease, look at the decisions you made that led you to this place, and learn to cope with certain stigmas surrounding HIV. Figuring out whom to trust requires questioning and discernment:

- Do you want to share this information with someone bound by confidentiality laws, such as a medical professional or counselor?
- Do you know someone personally who has dealt with this diagnosis or who is close to another individual with the disease?
- If so, is that person someone who tends to share things openly on social media 24/7?
- Will that individual judge you when he or she finds out you have HIV?

This process of questioning and evaluating is essential when figuring out whom to trust with sensitive information. The most important thing to remember in this process is that what you are sharing is for *your* purpose. This is about helping yourself, not fulfilling the wishes or expectations of others. So, if something needs to remain confidential, save it for someone who won't break that confidentiality. Again, examine your "why." Why do you want to share this information with someone, and why are you considering Person X, Person Y, etc.

It's important to trust your instincts. At Adams Recovery Center, we read each day from the "12 Steps to Self-Care," and one of the most important steps is trusting yourself. So, when you're considering sharing something with someone, ask yourself, *Does this person seem trustworthy?* Your instincts will take over, and that gut feeling will say, *No, this is something I don't feel comfortable sharing with them*, or,

Yes, my instincts tell me this person isn't going to be judging me or sharing this with anyone else.

Sometimes it can be hard to trust yourself in recovery, so let the behavior of others show you the way. Is someone saying things to you about other people or sharing other people's secrets? If so, then they'll probably do the same thing to you.

Of course, people are human, and sometimes they break your trust unintentionally. But most people genuinely mean well, and your instincts will guide you in making good decisions.

TRUSTING YOURSELF

Many times, people will come into our facility, and when we talk about trusting our instincts, they will say something like, "Well, I ended up here, so this is where my instincts took me."

We counter that with, "You are absolutely right, and you still ended up here because you knew you wanted to start a new, healthy life." Remember this: You have the power to trust yourself and to know that you, as an individual working toward long-term sobriety, can make solid decisions that can lead to lifelong healthy living.

You have more power than you think in every situation, and you deserve to trust yourself even if you've broken the trust of others in the past and even when others have broken your trust. Just because someone violated your trust doesn't mean there is no hope for you or your judgment. It goes back to that all-or-nothing thinking we discussed earlier. Often, individuals will see someone they highly respected break their trust, and they'll think, *Well, if they can't be trusted, then no one can—including me.* That's why you have to know in your bones that you are on the right path. If you're trusting the process, then you can trust yourself to make empowering decisions.

One technique to try is using self-talk reminders, such as "I can be trusted," "I am trustworthy," or "I have made mistakes in the past, but today I am honest and trustworthy." These reminders seem simple but can be very challenging because there are going to be people who remind you frequently that you have broken their trust in the past. The fact is, not everyone is going to forgive you for your past indiscretions.

You have to know in your own heart and mind that you are becoming a new, trustworthy person—regardless of what anyone else thinks.

Rebuilding the Trust of Others

Of course, it is important to acknowledge that you have violated the trust of others. In doing so, you might be asking, *How do I regain my loved ones' trust? Will I ever gain their trust back? Will there ever be healing from my past mistakes?*

The reality of the situation is that when trust is violated, some people will hold onto resentment, anger, and hostility. The good news is that you can work on regaining their trust in a variety of ways.

First and foremost, start with your actions. When it comes to trust, most people will agree that words have little power; your actions do all the talking.

So, start by being honest with the individual whose trust you have broken. It could be through a letter, phone call, or a face-to-face encounter. Be straightforward with the individual about what occurred and what you did. If you stole someone's jewelry and pawned it to support your addiction, tell her. Acknowledge what you did and let her know where you are today with regard to your addiction and making amends.

Honesty and candor go a long way in rebuilding trust. Be frank with your loved ones about where you are in your fight for sobriety and in your life in general. That will help them trust that you are on the right track and making progress. If you are struggling, be honest about that, too. Chances are, the people closest to you already know that, and you'll create more trust with honesty than by trying to hide your issues or pretending everything is okay.

Honesty doesn't mean you can't set boundaries with people. In fact, setting boundaries can be a great way to be honest! For example, you might choose to let your loved ones know up front what you're comfortable sharing at this point in your sobriety and what needs to remain private. If you let your mother know that you don't feel comfortable talking about your cravings, but you inform her that you want to go to a sober-support meeting or visit with a counselor, then you are being honest and trustworthy while protecting your privacy.

Now, here is the tough news: Mom might not believe what you say is going on. And that's where even more honesty comes in. To earn her trust, you might invite your mom to ride with you to the meeting, advise her that she can call your sober support or your counselor, or volunteer to take a drug screen upon your return. These kinds of things will let her know you are working a program. Patience goes hand in hand with honesty. Remember, your mom is looking out for your best interests, and because you didn't lose her trust overnight, you aren't going to regain it overnight either.

Another place to set boundaries is with people who are using or selling drugs. Simply put: Cut them out of your life. People in active addiction will not respect your boundaries or your priorities in maintaining health and sobriety. Furthermore, your family and friends won't take your recovery seriously if they feel you're not fully committed to moving beyond your unhealthy relationships.

Rebuilding trust—in yourself and with others—will take time. Be patient with yourself and your loved ones, and trust that the process is working.

• • • MELINDA'S STORY • • •

Melinda completed residential treatment in August 2016 and recognized that she had many problems related to her relationship with her mother. Melinda didn't want to move back in with her mother, but she also didn't want to go to sober living and have to start over again with a new group of women. Melinda's mother told her that if she relapsed, she would be kicked out of their home immediately. Melinda agreed that she must remain sober in the house.

A few weeks after the move, Melinda's mother told Melinda that she'd gone through her belongings because she was suspicious that her daughter was using heroin again. Melinda informed her mother that she was not using heroin and that she felt disrespected that her mom would go through her things. Melinda's mother said she would never be able to fully trust Melinda, and Melinda moved out in a rage. She said to her mother, "Since you think I'm high, I'm going to show you high."

Melinda relapsed and hasn't been heard from since. Though her story is very sad, it reflects the importance of respecting the time it takes to rebuild trust with friends and family members. It also serves as a reminder of the actions people in recovery might need to take to enable others to trust them again. We can only wonder where Melinda might be had she gone to sober living after treatment.

For Reflection

- Identify some individuals you feel you can trust. Why do you trust them? What qualities about them make them seem trustworthy?

_____

_____

_____

_____

_____

_____

_____

_____

- Name some people whose trust you would like to earn back. What are some things you can do to begin building bridges to them?

_____

_____

_____

_____

_____

_____

_____

_____

- When you think about honesty, how do you feel? Does the idea of honesty scare you? Challenge you? Make you feel free or at ease? What emotions are tied to the idea of being honest?

_____

_____

_____

_____

_____

_____

_____

_____

- Have you been clear in setting boundaries with your friends and family? What is working for you, and where do you need to be more honest about your limits and expectations?

_____

_____

_____

_____

_____

_____

_____

_____

- Recall a time when you trusted your gut and made a great decision, and then remind yourself of this example the next time you're tempted to doubt yourself.

  _____

  _____

  _____

  _____

  _____

  _____

  _____

  _____

CHAPTER THREE

Living with Integrity

Talking about addiction or individuals battling addiction usually includes words such as manipulation, dishonesty, and codependency. They're all negative terms that ultimately relate to someone's behavior—but not necessarily their character.

Treatment is a time not only to change behaviors but also to focus on restoring a person's core character so that person can live a better life, one with purpose. At the heart of character is integrity, and living with integrity is a key tenet of building a sustained sober lifestyle.

What exactly is integrity? At its most basic level, integrity means adherence to a code of moral values. For people in recovery, integrity has some very specific markers. For example:

- Around other people, and in a healthy environment, you're doing the next right thing. But when no one is around, are you the same person?
- Do you follow rules and laws?
- Are you honest?
- Do you care for others?
- Is there something greater that you are striving for?

A person who has integrity is always working toward building character, and that takes patience and a willingness to learn, become educated, and engage in self-reflection. It's one thing to learn something and quite another to put that knowledge into practice.

Education isn't necessarily about going to school, though that certainly can be part of it. Education is also learning from peers; seeking out experts such as therapists, counselors, doctors, and social workers who specialize in certain areas; and then reflecting upon the feedback given by those experts.

If you're working your program, chances are you have a gut feeling about whether you're building character and living with integrity. Here are some questions for a quick self-assessment:

- Are you meeting your goals and following through on your commitments?
- Are you being open and honest with your family about your current situation? If you are struggling, are you telling them or hiding it from them?
- Are you lashing out at others and then pretending everything is fine?

Losing integrity is a common issue among people entering recovery. During their treatment, they'll express that they've lost sight of who they truly are and that they did everything they swore they'd never do to their family and friends. They'll note that they stopped going to meetings and relapsed. They might even say they "couldn't talk to anyone," so they broke down and used.

All of that adds up to someone living without integrity and becoming a person he or she never expected to be. In some cases, disappointment over who they've become even leads to or prolongs use, as a means of numbing that pain.

In a therapeutic group setting, community members help one another by holding everyone accountable for the decisions they make. The goal is to make the same good choices privately that you make when others are watching.

Honesty Above All

Honesty is a key topic related to building integrity and character. Here's an everyday example: Let's say you're at your local fast-food chain and you give the cashier a twenty-dollar bill but she rings it up as a fifty. Are you going to be the individual who says, "No, I gave you a twenty"? Or are you the person who takes the extra change?

Something like this might not seem like a big deal, but let's think about it from a few different perspectives. First, that of the cashier: What might this mistake cost her? She might have to make up the difference from her own pocket—and that is definitely a big deal.

Now, let's look at the individual who took the additional money. Could that choice lead the person down a road of dishonesty? Many times, people in recovery recognize that their biggest issues started by not telling their loved ones the whole truth. Instead, they snuck by with half-truths. For example, a mom asks, "Are you back to doing heroin?" The addicted person says no—but fails to mention he is snorting cocaine. He justifies his half-truth by saying, "Well, she didn't ask if I was doing cocaine."

So, go back to the cashier at the fast-food chain. The justification for taking the extra change might be, "Well, she shouldn't have given me change for a fifty." That mentality is not one of a person living a life of honesty and integrity but rather of someone who is thinking mostly of self and not others.

Caring for others is something that needs to be practiced consistently for it to become second nature. Structure and consistency are crucial to all facets of sobriety. The concept is simple: If you say you are going to do something, then follow through on that commitment.

OPEN COMMUNICATION

Communication plays a major role in the commitment aspect of integrity. Asking peers and sober supports honest questions will help someone in recovery recognize her strengths and weaknesses related to consistency. Consider asking, "How do you think I am doing? How is my follow-through on things? Do you have any concerns?"

These questions will help build dialogue between you and your support system to enable you to recognize what areas still have room for improvement. This also will help you recognize the impact that you have on others, as well as the way you are presenting to others. Many times, people in addiction forget the major role they play in others' lives.

In addition to your family and friends, you're affecting the members of your recovery community and/or support groups. If you are attending meetings and being open and receptive to the concept of the program, you will help not only yourself but those around you, as well. Furthermore, building your character and acting consistently will inspire others to want to follow your lead, giving you a key role in your community. Even if you aren't aware of it, people are watching you, and how you act or react affects not only yourself but your community, as well. So, ask yourself: Do you want others to follow the example you're setting?

Another important point to remember: The people with whom you associate affect *your* integrity. If you are associating with dishonest people, are you also making excuses for these individuals? Too often in treatment, one client will say of another, "Yeah, I know she's not always honest with the staff, but she would never break my trust." Realistically, that's probably not true, and that means you're keeping yourself tied to lies and half-truths.

Honesty is vital to integrity. It's especially key to communicate honestly without seeking to be mean-spirited. Chances are you've learned in the past that being honest can be harmful. Learning to communicate honestly *and* productively is the challenge! For example, communicating honestly doesn't necessarily mean saying everything that's on your mind all the time. And honesty can be expressed lovingly and constructively. First, ask yourself, *Is what I am saying out of care and concern? Or do I have other motivations?*

Indeed, sometimes honesty will hurt or anger someone, but if there is a purpose behind the message, then the message can be of benefit to the individual or the group hearing it.

Finding a Balance

Something that will be of benefit to you is learning to say no. Many times, people will feel guilty telling someone that they cannot attend an important event or assist in a project of some kind. But remember: It is okay to say no. Think about follow-through. Does a person with integrity commit to an event or activity that she doesn't really believe in? Does a person with integrity commit to something and then not show up?

Many times, people new to sobriety will want to become "yes" people, because they believe they have missed out on so much that they have an obligation to meet every possible requirement. But taking on too much too soon can lead to stress and a struggle to follow through on important tasks, including self-care.

It might sound funny, but communicating honestly with yourself is crucial. For example, it can be easy to tell ourselves we will commit to something and then not follow through on the mission or goal because "I got too busy" or "I forgot." Ask yourself if those statements are true or if you actually avoided an event despite making a commitment.

And then, ask yourself why you made the commitment in the first place. Taking care of yourself and meeting your own needs is every bit as important as pleasing others, especially in early recovery.

Finding the right balance between caring for self and caring for others involves cultivating humility. A humble person will have a dedication to service, though what this service will look like for you could be very different than others might think. Service can include volunteering to work at a food pantry, volunteering for sober-support meetings, becoming a big brother—the list goes on and on.

A humble person also is eager to keep learning. Curiosity really didn't kill the cat! Find out what professionals think in areas that interest you. You could take classes at your library, attend therapy sessions, or check with your local community center to find a recovery coach.

Humility also comes from sharing our failures as readily as we share our successes. In doing so, we display our humanness and help others see how failures can be overcome. When you're able to describe to others how you got past your failures, you become a success story—and you help others do the same.

Making mistakes, growing, and coming back stronger are all part of leading a life of integrity.

Leo graduated from his first alcohol and drug treatment center in 1999. He was very proud of himself for completing thirty days and attending twenty-four classes in a corrective-thinking curriculum focused heavily on criminal thinking.

But Leo recognized in these courses that if he "faked it 'til he make-d it," he would be fine in the "real world."

Leo remained sober until 2016, when he began smoking pot. It had become legal for medical reasons in Arizona, where Leo recently had moved. Leo justified his marijuana use because his drug of choice was alcohol and he wasn't doing anything illegal.

After only two months of smoking pot, Leo began to drink at home alone. He thought nothing of it, because he was still not harming anyone and he had a legal prescription for marijuana. But it wasn't long before Leo was on a downward spiral with his drinking. He checked into a detox program, where he met a therapist and realized that he was not a "man of integrity"—he would say one thing but do another. Many times, Leo would tell people that everything was okay even though he was crumbling inside. He worked with this counselor for the next twenty-six weeks on how to develop integrity so his actions would match his words.

Leo recognized that although he was smoking marijuana legally, he wasn't taking it as prescribed; he knew he was just making an excuse to smoke a joint. Leo also recognized that he was lacking integrity in regards to his relationships; he was sponsoring people in sober-support groups just to look good to others rather than for the purpose of being a good group member. Leo admitted he had been mean-spirited toward his wife and had even cheated on her because she was "boring." He confessed to both his wife and the people he sponsored. Though the news was hard for all to handle and is still a work in progress, Leo knows this process is how he'll become a person with integrity.

For Reflection

- From one to five, with five being the highest, how would you rate your level of integrity? Do your private choices align with the choices you make publicly?

_____

_____

_____

_____

_____

_____

_____

- Think of someone you believe lives with integrity. What behaviors of theirs do you admire?

_____

_____

_____

_____

_____

_____

_____

_____

- How do you feel about saying no? Does it come easily, or do you struggle with overcommitting?

_____

_____

_____

_____

_____

_____

_____

_____

- Think about service to others. What does that mean to you? What are some forms of service that appeal to you?

_____

_____

_____

_____

_____

_____

_____

_____

_____

- Identify something you do consistently well and applaud yourself for it! Then, note an area in which you struggle to act or react consistently and write down three strategies for getting better.

_____

_____

_____

_____

_____

_____

_____

_____

CHAPTER FOUR

Navigating New Firsts

Do you remember the first time you rode a bike? How about the first time you drove a car? Some of our memories of major firsts are easy to recall. Other things that were once novel have become second nature, and we can't remember a time when we didn't know how to do them. In any case, most firsts are accompanied by some anxiety. If we didn't feel it ourselves, then our loved ones did as they stood by anticipating our success or failure. Think of the emotions of parents who wait for the bus on their child's first day of school. The child might not remember this big moment, but the parents probably always will recall the excitement and anxiety attached to their child boarding the bus and entering the world independently for the first time.

Early sobriety can feel very much like entering the world independently for the first time. Individuals in early recovery express anxiety, excitement, and fear associated with some of the firsts they will be facing: the first time they will parent without the aid of substances, the first time they will pay their own bills, the first time they will attend family events sober—even the first time they will date or have sex without using a substance to "take the edge off." The emotions attached to any of these events can feel overwhelming and might create a panicked state that can compromise an individual's self-esteem, creating a barrier to his or her recovery efforts. In this chapter, we'll look at ways to break down that barrier and stay on track through all of these firsts.

Let's start by recalling the first time you stopped using drugs and alcohol. You might have thought, *There is no way I can get through this. I don't know where to start. I don't know how I feel. What are feelings?* Having the clarity of experiencing feelings that have been suppressed through drug and alcohol use can leave you questioning how you will manage.

When we consider firsts, what we are really exploring is the unknown. Becoming comfortable with the uncomfortable is no easy task. This requires accepting the need for change and then following through with that change. Often, individuals with addiction issues express that they continued using drugs and alcohol simply because it was part of their routine. They had become comfortable in that routine until negative consequences became unbearable, prompting a need to do something different. Change is difficult. It challenges our perceptions. As you begin confronting your personal firsts, keep in mind the need for change and why it's important to you to engage in new behaviors in a sober lifestyle.

Also keep in mind that being uncomfortable is part of being human. Most individuals in active addiction have gotten used to instant gratification. One of the firsts they encounter in early recovery is recognizing that they will be all right even if they are uncomfortable. In fact, discomfort is necessary for growth. No one walks through life care-free, happy, and comfortable in every situation. In recovery, you learn that you no longer can avoid this truth by self-medicating with drugs and alcohol. You learn to do things differently.

So, what can you do if you feel overwhelmed and anxious about all these changes? You might have heard the saying, "One day at a time." For some, even this can be too much to think about. So, set a smaller goal: one hour at a time. And then to achieve that goal, identify what is creating your anxiety in the first place. Are the sources real or perceived? In other words, are these fears grounded in facts, or might you be projecting due to past experiences? Once you break down your thought processes, you will find it easier to reframe your thoughts, lessening the anxiety associated with the issue.

Here's a rough model:

- Break down each issue or event. Why is it important? What necessary change will it support or bring about?
- Explore why there is anxiety or fear attached to this issue.
- Assess whether the concerns are real or perceived.
- Set smaller goals that help minimize the fears attached to this issue.

WALKING THROUGH THE PROCESS

Breaking down the way you view "first" events will lessen the uncomfortable feelings you experience around them.

For example, let's consider the first time you attend a family event sober. Maybe there are family members who will be drinking or using other substances at this event. Perhaps you've attended these events under the influence in the past to relieve the anxiety that comes from communicating with your family. Maybe drinking is just part of your family's tradition. All of these factors can create anxiety. *Will I be able to participate in small talk? If there is drinking or using going on, will I want to do the same? Am I even able to be a part of family gatherings? What if some family members judge me and doubt my ability to change?*

As the fears pile up, make it a point to question each of them. Ask yourself if the fear is real or just perceived. If the fears are indeed real, then create a plan for dealing with the issues.

Rather than allowing yourself to become paralyzed with the emotions attached to this event, challenge yourself to become comfortable with the uncomfortable. Breaking down your thoughts about this event allows you to create new thought patterns that enable you to develop a plan of action.

For instance, if you know people will be drinking or using at the event, then you might choose to bring a sober support with you. If it's difficult to communicate with your family, you might have to practice the new communication skills you've learned in recovery about being honest and setting boundaries. You might have to endure family members who question your ability to change, accepting that as part of the process of recovery. You might even choose to create your own traditions and opt out of particular events.

Recognizing your strengths and weaknesses will help you select the right options for you. Protecting your serenity, your sense of well-being, should always remain your first priority. Anything that creates fear, anxiety, or tension might upset this sense, which is why it's important to take time during treatment to consider the firsts you'll face in your new life of sobriety.

Let's look at some other scenarios.

Beginning and Ending Relationships

Often, individuals express concern over beginning or ending relationships. Beginning new relationships without the aid of substances can spark feelings of fear and vulnerability, raise issues surrounding self-esteem, and create excitement, anticipation, and expectation. Ending relationships that might not support your sobriety can be equally emotional.

When considering starting a new relationship in early recovery, examine your motives for getting involved with someone. If you are learning how to navigate other important aspects of your life, such as working, attending meetings, repairing relationships within your family, and practicing self-care, are you ready to invest time and energy into another person? Could it be that you are searching for a distraction from these other areas of your life that might be overwhelming at times? Choosing to get into a relationship in early recovery can be risky, especially if you are not prepared to openly communicate your needs. Relationships involve another person whose emotions, needs, wants, and expectations must be considered. In other words, are you ready to engage with someone on this level without it affecting your serenity? If your last relationship was built on codependency and drug use, then beginning a new relationship sober can be a "triggering" event. It could create self-doubt, fear, and even resentment.

Self-doubt might come in the form of questioning your ability to have a good time without engaging in alcohol or drug use. It might leave you feeling fearful that you will not be able to open up or feel comfortable without that drink or drug that you felt took the edge off in the past. You might put too many expectations on yourself and the relationship as you are gaining self-respect and learning to commit to healthy boundaries. These expectations can create resentment if things do not go according to plan. Resentment will affect your serenity and might be a catalyst for negative self-talk and self-defeating behavior. All of that can increase the risk of relapse. As you can see, there are many aspects to consider. So, let's break it all down.

Start by honestly answering some potentially tough questions, such as: *Why am I considering involvement in a romantic relationship at this time? Am I creating a diversion because I am overwhelmed with other areas of my life? Am I able to commit to another person's needs while still caring for my own? How well am I managing the key areas of my life, such as work, meetings, self-care, and family?*

Based on those answers, you can set reachable goals and develop strategies for achieving them. If you realize you're starting a relationship because you're lonely, consider improving upon existing relationships with family and friends. If you come to see that your plate is full, you might consider waiting to start a relationship until you're more grounded in recovery. Being in a relationship can be draining. If you're already feeling overwhelmed, a relationship might be too much to take on and could compromise your progress.

Once you have broken down the details of your dilemma, you might see that making an impulsive decision based on emotions instead of logic might not have served you well in the past. Most importantly, you can set a plan to give yourself time to become comfortable with your present roles and responsibilities before taking on more that could create unnecessary anxiety. Don't forget that you're also forming a new relationship with yourself that needs time and space to develop.

When you become comfortable with the uncomfortable, you gain self-confidence and self-esteem. You learn to trust your instincts and identify your strengths and weaknesses.

You have less anxiety and fewer fears attached to beginning a new relationship when your confidence is strong. You are less likely to encounter expectations and resentment when you've allowed yourself the time to grow and learn how to emotionally navigate other important relationships in your life.

Along that line, you might need to end a relationship that could compromise your early sobriety and future goals. The process of assessing that situation is the same as the process you used to evaluate a potential new relationship. First, you must become comfortable with the uncomfortable by recognizing the need for change. Then, you can begin to question why there is fear and anxiety associated with this change. After all, if you know a relationship is toxic, why is there worry about letting it go? Remember, change challenges our perceptions, so what beliefs of yours are being called into question when you consider ending this relationship?

Let's work through the assessment process again.

First, ask yourself the tough questions and answer them honestly. For instance, if you are nervous about ending a relationship, is it because you're uncertain about your future and want to keep something familiar? Are you unsure how to create a new relationship if you let one go? By staying in a toxic relationship, are you really facing your fears? How can you grow in recovery if you are unwilling to let go of people, places, or things that made you feel comfortable in the past?

After you break down your feelings related to this scenario, you can identify why you have fears or anxiety and focus more clearly on whether these fears are real or perceived. You then can set achievable goals to question your fears and learn to recognize your strengths and weaknesses.

Early sobriety requires dedication to restructure the way you respond to situations. In addiction, you might have maneuvered through events with little or no regard as to how they made you feel. You might not have considered the consequences or outcomes of these events either. For the first time in a long time, you are recognizing the importance of acknowledging the thoughts and feelings associated with all you do, because you now understand the importance of protecting your serenity to maintain your sobriety.

• • • ELIJAH'S STORY • • •

Elijah entered treatment saying he had nothing in common with his peers because he'd had a "normal upbringing" and did not engage in criminal activities. He had not spent time in jails or other institutions. Elijah was feeling anxiety associated with seeking addiction treatment for the first time.

As Elijah progressed through the program, he continued to experience a series of firsts. For example, he began formulating genuine friendships that had nothing to do with using. He gave presentations in group sessions and began having assertive conversations with his peers and family for the first time. He experienced letting go of a friendship because the person was a potential threat to his serenity. That was something with which he'd struggled in the past, but for the first time, he was gaining the confidence to do what was required to protect his sobriety.

After completing the program, Elijah returned to share with other clients his story of more firsts in early recovery. He'd lost a family member and grieved without the crutch of a substance, even supporting other relatives instead of them needing to support him. He'd flown on an airplane without the aid of a substance to calm his fears, and he'd engaged with relatives who were less than enthusiastic about his journey in sobriety.

As Elijah continued to experience life with a new perspective, he recalled everyday firsts that he had not considered when he was in treatment. He described a moment at work when he was exposed to drugs and alcohol for the first time since leaving treatment. He noted the importance of breaking down that situation to examine what he was really feeling. He quickly felt a sense of relief and confidence as he was able to put this situation into a clearer context. He thought about what he had gone through when he was actively using drugs and alcohol and understood that the anxiety and fears he had were associated with past experiences of relapse. Although these concerns were real, he recognized that his perceived inability to stay the course in his sobriety was only imagined. Elijah then set the goal of recognizing his own strengths, recalling how hard he had worked to get where he was, and how using drugs or alcohol could take him away from all the goals he had set for himself. Elijah recognized that there could be several moments when he would be exposed to drugs and alcohol, but he could not let this detour him from earning a living.

Elijah was beginning to challenge himself by being comfortable with the uncomfortable. As Elijah continued navigating his first year of sobriety, he recognized that he had made it through the first sober birthday that he could remember, his first time dating sober, and, sadly, the first funeral he attended for a friend who did not survive his addiction. Through it all, Elijah expressed anxiety and excitement attached to these firsts. Though these events did create a sense of discomfort, Elijah became increasingly aware of his ability to get through such moments without using alcohol or drugs. That created a sense of empowerment, and his self-esteem grew. When asked what was the most important lesson he had taken from his first year in recovery, Elijah stated: "Something I have learned this past year is that it is not about what happens, it is about how you react to it. Balance is key."

There is no way of knowing what lies ahead in the first year of recovery. Many things could interrupt your serenity. Life is a beautiful series of ups and downs. Learning to manage both the good moments and the bad is crucial during your journey. There will always be challenges in early recovery associated with your firsts. As you become more comfortable with breaking down your thoughts and beliefs associated with those events, you will find you have less anxiety and more excitement attached to new experiences.

For Reflection

- When you consider your life in early recovery, what firsts—events or activities you'll experience sober for the first time—do you anticipate? How do you feel when you think about those things?

_____

_____

_____

_____

_____

_____

_____

_____

- Pick one of those issues—perhaps parenting sober or returning to the workforce—and break it down here. Examine why you feel anxious about the issue. What's at the root of that feeling?

_____

_____

_____

_____

_____

_____

_____

_____

- Now, ask yourself if the issues at the root of your feelings are real or just perceived based on your past experiences or other factors. If they are real, what are some strategies you can apply for navigating the challenges you'll face?

  _____

  _____

  _____

  _____

  _____

  _____

  _____

  _____

- Take a moment to think about change. Why are you making changes in your life? What goals can you set, even one hour at a time, to keep those changes on track?

  _____

  _____

  _____

  _____

  _____

  _____

  _____

  _____

- Identify a time when you made a difficult choice that allowed you to maintain your sense of serenity and well-being. Describe your process, and then take a moment to reflect with pride on your accomplishment!

_____

_____

_____

_____

_____

_____

_____

_____

CHAPTER FIVE

Avoiding Becoming Overwhelmed

Feeling overwhelmed is one of the most common reasons people cite for returning to drug or alcohol use after treatment. It's easy to become overwhelmed in sobriety, but fortunately there are many strategies for preventing this feeling.

Upon leaving treatment, many individuals jump full force back into their lives. They have missed so much because of their addiction—working, caring for the kids, paying bills, etc.—that they feel compelled to make up for lost time by doing everything all at once. That, however, just isn't realistic. As Elijah's story showed us in the previous chapter, balance is key!

To achieve—and stay in—balance, start by assessing the reality of the situation and asking some tough questions. If you're going back to work, will it be part time or full time? For many people, there is no choice but to go back full time. In that case, what's going to be the game plan at home? How will you schedule time for sober-support meetings, therapy sessions, and family activities?

It sounds simple, but buying a day planner, or using the planner on your phone, is essential. When you look at your calendar, have you left room for "me" time? If every second is blocked, then you're probably not leaving space for self-care. Don't forget how important it is to have time to yourself.

ASKING FOR HELP

Also remember that asking for help is perfectly okay. That can be a difficult concept for people in early recovery who believe doing things on their own is "the right way" to show that they're on track. But no one is Superman or Superwoman. A fear of asking for help is ingrained in our culture. Think back to the days before GPS. How many road trips ended up with wrong turns or begrudging stops at out-of-the-way gas stations—all because the driver didn't want to ask for help from the get-go? We want to say, "I got this," and seem in control, but the next thing you know, everyone in the car is headed down a long road to the middle of nowhere.

It's similar with sobriety; just as with a road trip, one wrong turn can lead to a detour that affects not only the driver, but his or her friends and loved ones, too. So, why not just ask for help? There are many factors, including a lack of education regarding addiction, a sense of weakness, and a perfectionist mentality.

In terms of education, many clients will tell us, "If I tell my mom I'm having cravings, she'll freak out." That's because many loved ones don't understand that cravings are natural and expected in sobriety. Without that education, the family member might immediately assume a relapse is occurring, and that assumption becomes a huge barrier to communication.

The perception of weakness is another issue, built into us by societal norms, even if unintentionally. For example, take the series of "Books for Dummies." These books are great assets; they help people learn things they might never have thought possible, and they can prevent someone from having to pay someone else to take care of an issue. This is wonderful! However, the title might make a person think, *Well, if I can't figure it out on my own, then I'm a failure.* When it comes to addiction, though, there is no one simple solution. There are many ways to find sobriety, and there isn't a book you can read (as much as we'd love for this book to be it) that will entirely "cure" your addiction. So, when you're feeling down, alone, stressed, or overwhelmed, reach out for help. It's the smart, responsible, and strong thing to do.

Now, let's look at that perfectionist mentality. What is it that has you wanting to do everything perfectly? Many times, this stems from childhood, a time when many clients say they were "never good enough" in school or sports. But as an adult, the perfectionist mentality can cause sadness, nervousness, and anger. People will tell us they are sad because they aren't living up to their full potential, nervous because they don't know what others will think of them, and angry because they just aren't good enough and they want to be the best. Instead, these questions can be more productive:

- Did you give your best effort in the given task?
- Did you consider the interests of others and yourself?
- Did you procrastinate? (We'll discuss this more shortly.)
- Are your expectations realistic?

If the answers to these questions reflect someone giving effort, showing empathy for others, managing time wisely, and setting realistic goals, then that person has done all he or she can to be successful. If the answers say otherwise, then it's an opportunity to look for ways to change behaviors and improve future outcomes. It's also important to remember that no one starts out at the top and no one is perfect, no matter how seemingly successful they are.

The Danger of Procrastination

So, let's pick up on the question about procrastination, which can easily lead to feeling overwhelmed. Often, people in early sobriety will put off important things, which leads to a stressful sense of urgency and a feeling of needing to take on many tasks all at once. Now, someone might not only feel overwhelmed, but he or she isn't set up to be successful— and that can be a blow to self-esteem.

Here's a common example we see with clients. Some individuals feel strongly about completing ninety meetings in ninety days after treatment. Though this might be a healthy and realistic goal for many people, it might not be for others. Many times, someone will think if she misses a meeting one day, then she needs to attend two the next day, essentially playing catch-up. This behavior not only exemplifies procrastination but also the perfectionist mentality. If a client is putting off something—a meeting, completing paperwork, seeing a doctor, etc.—we encourage her to identify how this could be detrimental to her long-term sobriety. How might putting off something important hinder her goals and create anxiety?

It is very easy to say, "Well, I will go to a meeting tomorrow," but too often the meeting tomorrow never comes. Structure is such a vital piece of sobriety, particularly in early recovery. Deviating from the routine can cause major problems. Though each person is unique, it's easy for most people to fall out of a healthy habit pretty quickly once the routine is compromised. Think of how many people you know (in recovery or not!) who "donate" to their local gyms with membership fees. They sign up, they go every day for a few weeks, and then take a day off. They'll go back…tomorrow. Now, a day off in and of itself is not such a bad thing, so long as the person is truly committed to this new healthy routine. It comes down to knowing and being honest with oneself and understanding what is needed to stay motivated.

If you're going to skip something that is part of your daily structure, first consider alternatives and then talk about your plans with someone you can trust to be open and honest with you.

Creating a Healthful Schedule

Almost anyone in recovery is going to feel overwhelmed at some point—it's natural and expected. So, the key is to learn ways to manage that feeling. Step one: Learn to say no. Saying no can be challenging, but it's the best way to avoid taking on too much. If you look at your planner and your week is booked, then start saying no to others so you can make time for yourself. Yes, it might hurt someone's feelings or cause you to feel bad for a moment. But consider: At the end of the day, your serenity and sobriety are far more important than a lunch, a shopping trip, or a night out with friends.

Two other important factors are sleep and nutrition. Sleep is crucial to maintaining your mental health. Give yourself ample time to fall asleep and stay asleep without interruption. Also, examine what and when you are eating. If you find yourself eating at odd times and choosing not-very-healthy options, blood-sugar imbalance could be contributing to some of the sense of being overwhelmed. In our treatment centers, clients eat breakfast, lunch, and dinner at the same time every day to build a healthful routine. Stability is imperative, and that includes stability in your sleep patterns and your eating habits.

Lastly, set aside some quiet time. In our centers, we reserve thirty minutes a day for quiet time. Television and mindless banter can be distracting. True quiet time allows you to read, reflect, engage in a creative project, or even meditate. Many times, the brain is on constant "go," and having some time to reflect can provide peace. Peace doesn't just happen; it is a practice. Even though Western societies love to be on the move, it is okay to sit back and enjoy life by just observing.

Be aware of who you are and where you are, and get in touch with your inner self.

• • • TABITHA'S STORY • • •

Tabitha completed residential treatment in early 2017, having recognized that she had a perfectionist mentality and needed to accept that she makes mistakes. Upon moving to sober living, Tabitha became one of the most popular ladies in the program. She found stable employment, got shared parenting of her sons, and attended church services every Wednesday and Sunday.

As time progressed, Tabitha's popularity became a major problem for her. She often had many friends asking her to do different things during the week on top of her other responsibilities. Tabitha slowly began to spend more time with her friends than she did with her sons, and she began missing church services regularly.

Tabitha eventually relapsed. But back in treatment again, she recognized that she was so focused on making other people happy, she wasn't considering what her busy schedule was doing to her sobriety. Tabitha looks back now and believes that had she been able to say no and focus on her responsibilities, she would not have started using cocaine again.

Tabitha has become involved in weekly yoga classes, attends outpatient alcohol and drug counseling, is back to attending church services, and spends the weekends with her boys. She says the biggest thing she has learned is that it is okay to say no to people; that feeling is much better than the overwhelmed feeling she had from saying yes to everyone. Tabitha says structure has been the most important piece to her long-term sobriety.

FOR REFLECTION

• How balanced is your lifestyle currently? Are you making as much time for yourself as you are for others? Where is there room for improvement?

_____

_____

_____

_____

_____

_____

_____

• Identify one thing to which you could say no more often (or permanently) to create more space in your schedule for quiet time.

_____

_____

_____

_____

_____

_____

_____

_____

- What's something on which you procrastinated recently? Did you ultimately get the task done? How did procrastination affect your serenity and the outcome of the task?

  _____

  _____

  _____

  _____

  _____

  _____

  _____

  _____

- When was the last time you asked for help? How did you feel when you sought assistance? What was the result of your request?

  _____

  _____

  _____

  _____

  _____

  _____

  _____

  _____

- What are some things you enjoy doing by yourself to relax? How much time have you carved out for them in your schedule?

  _____

  _____

_____

_____

_____

_____

_____

_____

CHAPTER SIX

Managing Family Dynamics

Whether you yourself are in recovery or the family member of someone who is recovering, the way you interact with one another must change. Many family members say, "I just want my old son or daughter back," and even individuals in recovery might say, "I just want my old life back," or, "I just want to be the person I was before all this started." But that is a destructive thought process. When it comes to treatment and recovery, the whole process is about change. To move forward, there can be no going back.

If you're wishing for the way things used to be, take a moment to remember what went wrong and consider why. Were you really happy back then? What issues existed that led to the addiction in the first place?

Regardless of how a person comes into addiction, the reality is that he and his family must move forward by dealing with who the person is now. Drug and alcohol addiction changes people. It changes a family's dynamic, as well. Trust has been broken, communication has been compromised, and many family members and people in recovery have much denial attached to all of it.

Individuals in recovery might seek to protect their family members by saying their families have always supported them and taking the blame for all the family's dysfunction. Merriam-Webster defines dysfunctional as "abnormal or unhealthy interpersonal behavior or integration within a group." When individuals in recovery try to protect their family members, it is likely due to guilt and shame they feel for their role in the family dysfunction. But they did not create it alone.

Every family is unique. Some express themselves openly, without hesitation, whereas others adopt the "don't ask, don't tell" policy to keep the peace when problems arise.

As family members struggle to understand why someone in their family is plagued by addiction, they might blame themselves as well. They might take on the role of defending their loved one's behaviors. In fact, some family members are so dedicated to taking the blame or blaming others that they fail to recognize that the person with the addiction is still suffering and is unable to communicate her needs openly and honestly.

In this chapter, we'll look at some of the barriers to communication, explore methods for breaking those barriers, and provide hope that even though the road is difficult, it absolutely *can* lead to the positive changes you want to see.

COMMUNICATION CHALLENGES

In a perfect world, family communication would be effortless. Everyone would be mindful of what others might be thinking or feeling. There would always be time to talk, and all conflicts could be resolved quickly over a dinner, with no raised voices, discouraging remarks, or hurt feelings. Reality is much different.

Communication in many families is surface-level at best. The culture has produced a generation of text-savvy communicators. So, when serious issues arise, many families struggle with expressing their needs or feelings. Whether it's out of fear about how someone might respond or out of frustration with different perspectives among family members, communication becomes a challenge for many trying to resolve family conflicts and dysfunction.

Of course, addiction creates many barriers to effective communication. Whereas some individuals might openly discuss with their co-workers and friends the struggles they face about allowing their daughter to wear makeup or accepting their son's new romantic interest, those same people rarely talk to their support systems about family stories related to addiction.

This might be due to the stigma attached to addiction. The fear of being judged by others or labeled as "*that* family" often leads to isolation and despair for many family members.

The fear of exposing the addict or alcoholic's behaviors might be one of the many reasons why communication becomes more difficult. If you are covering up, minimizing, justifying, or rationalizing what your loved one is doing to himself and the family, you are fostering relationships based on denial. When you are in denial about anything, no real changes can be made. You must accept what is taking place if you're going to resolve the problem.

Trust and Empathy

Trust and empathy also can be communication barriers created by addiction. As with fear of exposure, there might be hesitation to trust or empathize with the individual who is in early recovery. Individuals who were in active addiction have exhausted not only themselves but their family members, as well. They have used manipulative tactics to gain sympathy for their continued use and have broken the trust with their support systems in the process.

Trust and empathy are two-way streets. The person in recovery must trust that her family members will no longer enable her. She must trust that her family will allow honest communication and keep open minds about the changes she is attempting to make. She also must trust herself to make good choices in recovery while having empathy for herself and for others who have been affected by her behaviors.

Rebuilding trust is something that will, and should, take time. To put complete faith in everything the recovering individual says or does immediately actually might compromise the person's sobriety. Addiction is more than being dependent upon alcohol and drugs; it's about behaviors, as well. For example: In the past when the individual followed through on something he or she had promised, it may have come with a "reward"—a hit of the person's drug of choice. Individuals in early recovery must learn that the real reward is a better life filled with honest relationships built on respect and effective communication. Trust takes time, and as long as both parties are open-minded and willing to work together on boundaries and respect, healthy communication will foster that trust once again.

Empathy is much different from sympathy. Sympathy is feeling sorry for someone, and it can cause family members to give an addicted person money, fix his or her problems, or lie to others on their loved one's behalf to maintain some sense of peace within the family. This is enabling, and it does not promote healthy communication. Sympathetic acts might resolve an issue for the moment, but they are ineffective in the long run.

To empathize means to put yourself in another person's shoes. Looking at how the individual in early recovery might feel can help you develop a sense of the appropriate way to deal with certain situations. If your loved one appears to be struggling, remind her how far she has come, recognize her strengths, and never minimize her feelings. Remember that you do not need to fix anything for her. Support looks much different when you learn to communicate openly and honestly without expectations from either party.

THE NEED FOR HOPE

Family members who are dealing with someone with addiction often give up and lose hope. They might feel they have exhausted all means of expressing concern for their loved one, from being understanding and trying to empathize with their loved one's struggles to pleading and bargaining for change. Eventually, some family members might become angered by their loved one's continued promises to change and the failure to follow through on these promises.

During this time of detachment, some family members might even fantasize about a "better life" without their addicted loved one. Just as an active addict or alcoholic expresses a desire to "end the pain," family members who have exhausted all their energies, often with little support, may experience that same desire for an ending to relieve their worries and struggles.

One mother who was desperate for change stated: "I am so tired of all of this. I even prayed that she would die so that she would not be in pain anymore and I wouldn't have to worry every day what is going to happen to her."

This mother was clearly overwhelmed. She had done all she believed she could to help resolve her daughter's addiction issues. But there was one resolution left unexplored: the determination to learn how to effectively communicate and set healthy boundaries. She and her daughter had spent years talking *at* each other instead of talking *to* each other. The mother would express what she wanted or needed from her daughter, and her daughter would hide her feelings and concerns so as not to upset her mom. The daughter was aware that she was "letting her mother down," as her mother had to take on the responsibility of raising her daughter's child. The daughter was often incarcerated or in treatment over the course of several years, so she understood that she had become a burden to her family. She did not dare to disagree with her mother's directives for fear that she would be completely excluded from her child's life. She was unable to express her true feelings. As a result, she continued to carry the emotions and low self-esteem that had plagued her since childhood. That meant she continued to harbor the feelings and behaviors that contributed to her addiction.

When the daughter entered treatment once again, her mother had lost hope that there could be any real, substantial change. The mother would come to the visitations with her daughter's child and say things such as, "You need to stop putting us both through this," and, "I need you to come home and get a job, so you can help pay for your kid. This is just wasting time!" The daughter felt hopeless; she wanted to change but felt she had little encouragement to do so. She expressed how her mother and child might both be "better off without her." She had tried to talk to her mother about how she was feeling, but her mother had reached a point of frustration and anger that left her unable to trust that this time would be any different. She was convinced that this was just another excuse by her daughter to avoid growing up and taking responsibility for her child.

Unfortunately, both mother and daughter got their "wish." The daughter died of an overdose shortly after leaving treatment. She was unable to process all the guilt and shame she had lived with throughout the course of her life. She was unable to communicate her feelings with the most important people in her life. Everything she knew about recovery had little impact on her because she was unable to build the self-confidence and self-esteem that could help her sustain long-term sobriety.

The mother was heartbroken. Of course, she never really wanted her daughter to die. She was left with the same unanswered questions she'd had over all the years her daughter had struggled. *Why did she turn to drugs and alcohol? Was it something I did? What was missing in her life? Why wasn't her child enough reason to stay sober?* This was followed by more anger and blame.

This is an example of how important communication can be for both family members and individuals in recovery. Without both parties keeping an open mind and learning about addiction, codependency, enabling, and ways of setting healthy boundaries and communicating, rarely does the outcome change.

STRATEGIES FOR SUCCESS

Individuals struggling with addiction must let go of the emotions and feelings associated with their drug and alcohol use. They must feel they can express these feelings and emotions openly and without judgment. They must release the guilt and shame attached to the behaviors they've displayed, and they must feel supported in doing this. Early sobriety brings clarity. Individuals who have struggled with alcohol and drug use are well aware of how much their addiction has cost them and their families emotionally, physically, and often financially.

Even though family members have given their support to their loved ones in the past, they must now evaluate how this support has either helped or hurt the situation. Family members might have many of the same struggles with letting go of their emotions and feelings as does the drug addict or alcoholic. They also must feel that they can express these thoughts and feelings openly and without judgment. They might need to let go of the guilt and shame they have attached to their perceived role in their loved one's addiction. Most importantly, they must recognize that even though this has cost them in the past, they cannot give up hope: hope for a better life for the individual struggling, as well as hope that they might someday work as a family unit again. Hope is the one thing that can foster the positive communication that is so crucial to individuals in sobriety and family members alike.

That said, although hope is key to healthy communication, hoping and wishing for something do not create change.

When considering all the barriers to healthy communication, you might find yourself struggling with where to begin. There is a saying in recovery: "All you have to change is everything." That's no big deal, right?

Family members might be expecting many changes from the individual who is battling addiction, but what changes are they willing to make to increase the chances of success? One important change to consider might be to educate yourself on addiction issues. It's hard to seek support if you are battling stigmas attached to your loved one's addiction. The more you learn about the origins of addiction, the more you might feel comfortable discussing your feelings openly with your loved one and with outside support systems. Outside support gives family members an opportunity to step back and hear another perspective that could help them, much the way a person in recovery has sponsors, meetings, or counselors helping him or her.

Another change that family members might consider is understanding and recognizing the differences between healthy and unhealthy boundaries. Boundaries are not meant to punish or shame an individual; rather, they are set in place to protect each person's rights and clearly define what is or is not acceptable by the person setting the boundary. Boundaries should be mutually understood. Boundaries should also be reasonable and flexible. Healthy boundaries must always come with consequences, and these consequences must be enforced. If you have set a boundary but you routinely allow another person to cross it, who bears the blame? If you do not follow through on consequences, what you are really saying is, "These are just words, and you can ignore my feelings and wishes." That is a very unhealthy way of communicating. It sends mixed messages, and no change will occur. Much of the inability or unwillingness to set healthy boundaries is attached to codependency. As family members and people in recovery will attest, once they discover what codependency really is, there is no denying how that dynamic played a part in the addicted individual's continued use.

As with anything worth pursuing in life, recovery requires work and education. If you're struggling with addiction—whether yours or someone else's—remember that there is hope for better days for all involved. Use this hope to help you pursue a new way of understanding and communicating with your loved one. Do not forgive and forget too quickly, but allow yourself to let go of the past and move toward a better future. It's all right to be angry or frustrated by the situations that are occurring. What is not all right is to dwell on those feelings. That's just wasted energy. Recognize that people don't get to the extremes of their addiction independently; they have had some help along the way. Someone has enabled them, allowed them to manipulate, become codependent on them, or simply turned their head, wishing and waiting for something to change.

When considering more effective communication, think of all the things this entails. This means becoming mindful of what the other person might have going on before entering a serious discussion. In other words, empathize. Ask the other person if he or she has time to talk. If not, then set a time that is mutually agreed upon. This allows the other person to be prepared that something important is about to take place. Think about how you might feel if someone were to approach you right before you were getting ready to walk out the door for work. The conversation might be rushed, you might not be receptive to what the other person is saying, and your focus might be on ending the conversation so you can get out the door. This is often how miscommunication begins. The other person could feel offended because you did not give him the time to fully express what he wanted to say. That might not have been your intention, and you might feel upset by his lack of understanding. Something as simple as scheduling a time to talk can be the start of better communication.

If, for whatever reason, the person does not show up at the agreed-upon time, this is a great opportunity to start setting boundaries. The next time you encounter this person, you might start from the beginning by asking him if he has time to talk. If he says no again, explain how this makes you feel and tell him that until he is ready to have a serious conversation, then perhaps communication should be limited.

Once a person is engaged in the conversation, try to use "I" statements. Do not approach someone with "You did this…" or "When you do that…" These types of statements are accusatory and will cause a person to become defensive, halting communication efforts. Instead, try saying, "I feel upset when I see this…" or "I worry when…" You can see how differently these statements make you feel. People are more receptive to and less likely to disagree with your feelings versus your observations.

After expressing your concerns and describing how something makes you feel, allow for a response. Remember, communication requires active listening. The goal is to talk *to* someone, not *at* someone. The other person's feelings are just as important as yours, even if you do not agree with them. Allowing the other person to be heard fosters trust and honest dialogue.

Another point to remember is your tone of voice. Do not speak over someone or speak loudly. Body language is also important. You can tell how your words are affecting others by looking at how they physically react to them. For example, if they cross their arms, slouch, or avoid eye contact, they might be feeling defensive. This might help guide the way you are addressing an individual.

Most importantly, don't expect to "win" an argument or discussion. It's all right to agree to disagree. When you go into a discussion feeling righteous, you lose all perspective on how the other person might feel. There does not need to be a winner in the conversation. Conversing is merely an opportunity to have your feelings heard. How another person responds is not your responsibility.

As noted earlier in this chapter, in a perfect world, communication would be effortless. But that just isn't reality. We must strive to communicate better with our loved ones, making sure they feel encouraged, safe, accepted, and understood. Even if you do not fully understand addiction, you can empathize with the struggle. When you educate yourself on all the issues that surround addiction, such as codependency, enabling, boundaries, and healthy communication, what you are really saying to your loved one is, "You are worth it. I'm trying to understand and make a difference." You are also recognizing the need to change some things yourself.

If you are reading this, you already have identified how important communication and education are. Do not give up hope that you might reconnect with your loved one on a healthier level. Whether you are a person still struggling with addiction, someone in recovery, or a family member or friend of someone who has addiction issues, remember that hope, backed by change and effective communication, might be the strongest, most effective tool you will have in this fight.

• • • JESSICA'S STORY • • •

Jessica had spent years isolated in her addiction. After several attempts at sobriety, she decided to enter treatment once again. She struggled at first to open up and discuss any issues with her counselor. Instead, she continued bottling her feelings, which reinforced her negative self-talk and low self-esteem.

After weeks of surface-level communication, her counselor encouraged Jessica to really look at why she was in treatment and the reasons why treatment had not worked for her in the past. Jessica broke down crying as she disclosed how she had not spoken with her daughter in over ten years. She did not feel worthy of recovery. She had spent years isolated from the people she loved, continuing to tell herself that they were better off without her. There were moments over the years when she had done well, but they were short-lived. Each time she had clarity in her life and was doing the right things, she would convince herself that too much time had passed, and she didn't know where to begin to rebuild the trust and relationship with her daughter.

Jessica was convinced that abandoning her daughter all those years ago was one of the main reasons she could not be successful in recovery. Every time she was doing well, the guilt and shame she felt became overwhelming. She did not tell anyone about it out of fear of judgment. She had learned to minimize, justify, and rationalize why it was okay to keep living her life irresponsibly and chaotically.

Until this moment with her counselor, Jessica had never expressed to her family or friends how deeply not being a part of her child's life had affected her. By beginning to have genuine discussions with her counselor, Jessica was able to let go of her guilt and shame. She decided that she had been avoiding a major area of her life for far too long and was ready to contact her daughter.

Jessica worked closely with her counselor and peers on ways she would do this. Through a phone call? Through a letter? She was unsure where to start. She continued to work with people with whom she was developing trust and then spoke with what she thought was a supportive family member. This family member had stood by Jessica for years during her absence in her daughter's life. She would tell Jessica things like, "It's not your fault," and, "I will let her know." This person had served as a go-between for Jessica and her daughter for years.

But when Jessica finally decided to reunite with her daughter and needed her phone number to do so, this family member quickly became angered. She was mad that Jessica was independently reaching out. She felt vulnerable because she did not know where she fit into the relationship anymore. She had become dependent on "fixing things" for Jessica, and Jessica's independence felt like a threat to her now.

Jessica spent several weeks patiently communicating her intentions to this third party and letting this person know that she was very much appreciated and needed, but the role she played in Jessica's life had to change. Jessica began setting healthy boundaries and continued assertive and empathetic communication with this person. The third party ended up giving Jessica the information she needed to arrange a phone call with her daughter. Jessica had learned the importance of clear boundaries, empathy, assertiveness, and letting go of expectations long before she attempted to make her first call to her now-adult daughter.

When she did make the call, her daughter was very receptive and understanding, agreeing to continue working on communication and possibly to arranging a visit that might begin the healing process. As time went by, Jessica became more comfortable calling her daughter. Their relationship was getting stronger each week, and Jessica continued to open up about other factors that had created barriers to her recovery in the past. As they grew together, Jessica became stronger in her recovery.

She even discussed the importance of communication in the speech she made when graduating treatment. Through teary eyes, Jessica expressed how important her recovery journey was to her and her child. She shared the story of how they had reunited and how much it meant to her that they had found each other again. When Jessica's daughter appeared in the doorway, the room erupted in applause. Jessica's daughter had no idea what had been said previously.

Jessica looked at her daughter, introduced her to the crowd, then walked over and hugged her. Her daughter showed up to support her mother for completing this first step in sobriety. The daughter expressed gratitude and hope for a continued relationship with her mother.

Jessica went on to sober living and continued to work on her relationship with her daughter. Jessica allowed herself to trust that she was worthy of this relationship and that her daughter could forgive her. Jessica's daughter continued to hope that her mother would put the effort into their relationship and be a part of her life. The two of them together discussed setting healthy boundaries and letting go of expectations; they talked about their fears, their feelings, and their faith.

The key word here is "discussed." They communicated openly and honestly with each other, learning that there did not have to be a so-called winner in the discussion. It took time, and the time they spent together was genuine and something they both appreciated. Jessica admits that she occasionally engages in self-defeating thoughts about how she "waited so long and lost so much time" with her daughter. But Jessica states: "The difference now is I recognize that I can't go back, but I can always move forward. The way our relationship is now is all because I had to learn how to trust and respect myself and her."

FOR REFLECTION

- What are the primary communication challenges your family faces?

_____

_____

_____

_____

_____

_____

_____

_____

- Do you understand the difference between sympathy and empathy? Write down an example of a time when you felt sorry for someone and compare it to a time when you truly put yourself in someone else's shoes.

_____

_____

_____

_____

_____

_____

_____

_____

- How hopeful do you feel right now about the addiction issues in your life? Even if it's hard, write down three reasons not to lose hope.

_____

_____

_____

_____

_____

_____

_____

_____

- Think about someone with whom you need to have an important conversation. What are five "I" statements you could use to help make your point without being accusatory?

_____

_____

_____

_____

_____

_____

_____

_____

- When have you been part of successful communication around a difficult topic? What took place that enabled things to go well?

_____

_____

_____

_____

_____

_____

_____

_____

CHAPTER SEVEN

Handling the Holidays

Holidays can be challenging for everyone, but for individuals in recovery, they can be especially difficult. Holidays are meant to be a time of celebration, family, and friends, as well as a chance to take a break from the day-to-day stresses of life. When a person is in recovery, however, holidays can create new stress, including conflict and the temptation to join in the festivities in the same way he or she might have done in the past. Individuals in recovery also might be struggling with forming new relationships with family and friends. This might leave them feeling vulnerable, wondering how they will participate in holiday events where alcohol or drug might be present. This chapter will explore some of the challenges that individuals in recovery might face, along with ways to alleviate some of the stress that might accompany these times of celebration.

STICKING TO A SCHEDULE

First, let's talk about structure. It is extremely important for individuals in recovery to develop some sense of structure. During active use, people do not keep schedules consistently. Many express how they were just living day to day, their schedules dependent upon their use. Much of their time was spent pursuing their drug of choice, figuring out ways to pay for it, using, and planning to use again. This was the closest thing to structure many can recall. In recovery, one of the first things learned is how to set a schedule based on self-care and personal priorities. It's important to focus on the seemingly simplest things, such as getting up each day at a set time, bathing, getting to work, caring for family, and attending meetings. A set schedule protects a person in early recovery by lessening the amount of down time when it might be tempting to fill the void with unhealthy choices.

The structure provided through scheduling becomes a new way of life for a person in recovery, and the slightest alteration can be a challenge. Something as simple as sleeping in one day can have a person in early recovery feeling anxious and out of sorts. So, holidays can become problematic when the normal schedule is interrupted. Instead of a regular work day, there might be an atypical day off. To someone in recovery, this down time can be dangerous. He might recall what he used to do on the holidays. He might just feel bored. As it has been noted, two things consistently lead to individuals using again: bad relationships and boredom.

Mixed with the emotions that holidays can bring, boredom can be devastating for a person in recovery. Sticking as closely as possible to the usual routine is good protection. Try to adjust your work schedule to meet the holiday demands. If you do not have to work, try to remain consistent with your day, adhering as much as you can to the plan that you have become accustomed to: wake up at the same time, eat a healthy breakfast, etc. When you do have to alter your schedule, remember to include sober activities that you can enjoy along with the regular self-care you have been doing each day.

Emotional Highs and Lows

Strong emotions are another possible holiday pitfall. Holidays have a way of causing us to recall certain times in our lives, both good and bad. The emotions tied to those memories can create a lot of anxiety and depression. Whether it's a longing for the "good ol' days" or dread of the holiday due to past painful events, the emotions can feel overwhelming to a person in recovery. In some cases, the holidays might cause someone to remember times spent with special people who are no longer in their lives for various reasons. It can be hard to make it through without someone important. Grieving—whether a death or a lost relationship—at a time when people are celebrating can feel completely deflating. As a result, someone in recovery might try to wear a mask of happiness around peers, family members, or co-workers when in reality she is mourning the loss of someone dear or adjusting to creating a new tradition without a loved one. This sort of mourning also applies to individuals who have had to give up some of their favorite people or places to maintain their sobriety. During the holidays, dealing with grief and loss can create a sense of loneliness that was once numbed by drugs and alcohol. Heightened emotions can lead to a desire to find comfort and relief. This is when some people convince themselves that having just one drink or using just one more time will be okay.

Instead, it's vital to find new, healthier ways of dealing with grief, such as speaking with someone, going to meetings, or helping others who might be struggling. Strategies learned in recovery also are key: Thought-stop techniques, breathing techniques, and meditation can help lessen the internal struggles. This is an especially good time to seek out sober supports or go to a meeting to be in the company of others who might be feeling the same way.

Some emotions attached to the holidays stem from expectations—expectations you might put on yourself or expectations that might come from others. People in recovery might feel as though they have short-changed some of their loved ones in the past due to their addiction. Now sober, they feel they have to make up for lost time. They might feel as though they need to provide the perfect gift to a loved one even if finances dictate otherwise. They might feel as if people at a party are expecting them to act or be a certain way. If in the past they did not attend family events due to addiction, they might feel obligated to be there now. This amounts to a perfect storm of self-defeating thoughts and behaviors. Expectations can lead to resentment, and that compromises serenity. Expectations also create an opportunity for guilt and shame to re-emerge, fostering a risk of relapse. The focus must remain on sobriety! If attending an event might be too stressful, then respectfully decline or make arrangements to share time with special individuals in a more suitable atmosphere.

However, do not use this as an excuse to isolate either, especially if isolation was a behavior you used during active addiction. Knowing that your serenity must always come first, you might find it comforting to remind yourself that you are not responsible for how others think or feel.

Other challenges related to holidays are a hurried pace and increased contact with society. Work-related parties, traffic, and crowds in stores all can lead to long waits and short fuses for people who are already struggling with day-to-day issues. Anger and resentment are great motivations for relapse. Many recovering individuals recall that they were angered or felt wronged in some way before choosing to take that first drink or use that drug again. Only later do they recognize that their anger and resentment were just excuses for them to use. Unfortunately, around holidays, many people are looking for just that—an excuse to use.

Emotions coupled with external stressors might seem unbearable, but if you stop, take a deep breath, and remember that this is just another day, you can gain control over the impulsive thoughts you're experiencing. You can stop and recall the coping skills you've learned and use this as an opportunity to put them to work.

Family-related Stress

Coping with family members is a huge element to any holiday. Families, even supportive ones, can create much anxiety. At holidays, you might encounter some family members whom you have not seen in a while, plus some you might rather avoid. Making small talk with these individuals can be quite daunting. Many families use time together to sit, talk, and drink. For someone in recovery, such an event can feel like an eternity. This is why it is so important to plan ahead. Perhaps you can bring your "accountabili-buddy," that person who understands what you're going through and can give you a way out while holding you accountable for your actions and reactions. You also can plan other things to do in the nearby area, such as seeing a movie or going to a meeting, to help reduce the amount of time you have to spend sitting around.

Some families use these get-togethers to vent past grievances when everyone is a captive audience. Remember that you do not have to indulge in this behavior. Stay away from drama and negativity. Even if it's between Uncle Bob and your mom, it can be toxic to you. Some family members might be looking for the opportunity to bring up your past. For example, now that you are sober, you can recall the money you owe so-and-so—that's the logic of some family members. This is a time to practice some of the self-care you've learned in early recovery, recalling instructions such as "Don't be a people pleaser" or "Let go of what you can't control." Be assertive, using "I" statements and being clear about how you feel, to communicate effectively with family members.

As with any social event, if it feels too overwhelming, then simply opt out and create your own holiday tradition. The goal is to get through this day or days with your sobriety and serenity intact.

New Year's Eve

Let's look at one holiday in particular that may spark anxiety: New Year's Eve. You don't have to be in recovery to feel anxious about this holiday! A new year might bring new expectations. Failed resolutions from previous years can spark negative self-talk. You might say to yourself, *What's the point? Why will this year be any different? It always ends the same.* New Year's Eve has a way of creating both extreme excitement and deep sadness. You might be excited to move forward and have new opportunities in the upcoming year while feeling regret for what was not completed during the past year.

Another aspect to consider when moving into a new year might be that not everyone will be joining you in this upcoming year. One thing often said to individuals in early recovery is that not everyone is meant to go on with you in this next part of your journey in life. Simply put, you will have made clear choices to let go of toxic relationships that do not support your recovery efforts. Yet during a New Year's celebration, you might feel a renewed sense of loss. Even if you lost someone years ago, New Year's Eve has a haunting way of reminding us of just what we are leaving behind and who cannot or will not be part of our lives moving forward.

The pressures of being with someone special to ring in the new year can lead to isolation and despair, especially if that someone is no longer with you due to death or the choice to move forward without him or her. New Year's is a time of rebirth, an opportunity to begin fresh. If you have given up a toxic relationship and find yourself alone going into the new year, this could be a very stressful time for you, especially if one of the things you are working on is codependency and enabling. You might be facing the reality of not only moving forward without drugs and alcohol but of doing so independently, and that could have you feeling very alone or defeated.

As with all holidays, one suggested tool to alleviate anxiety is to recall the reason for the season. New Year's is a time for starting over with a clean slate, and this is exactly what you are doing. You are learning to navigate through the holidays and celebrations without the baggage of old coping mechanisms and hurtful belief systems. You are bringing new values into your new year.

• • • CARL'S STORY • • •

Carl entered into a recovery program, reluctant and arrogant. Although he struggled (as many do) in the beginning, Carl developed a sense of pride about his program and his recovery. He would get very excited as he looked to his future and saw how his growth would benefit him and his son once he left treatment. He was working on self-esteem, boundaries, guilt, and shame. He was excelling in his program and becoming a leader among his peers. He showed compassion and concern for others, which was huge for him, because he had been very self-centered and critical of others when he first entered treatment.

As the holidays approached, a change began to occur with Carl. He was not sharing in groups as much, did not appear to care one way or another about his peers, and was becoming cynical and anxious. He was very much resembling the person he was when he entered treatment. Carl then disclosed why he was acting the way he was. He revealed that he had been incarcerated during Christmas for the past three years. He had promised his son the previous New Year's that he would not miss another Christmas with him, and Carl was anxious because he knew he was only halfway through his program and if he stayed, he would not be able to keep his promise to his son.

Both staff and peers challenged his thoughts as he expressed that "no matter what," he was going to be home at Christmas with his son, "even if it cost him his program." The fact was, Carl was on probation. Leaving treatment would have violated his terms, causing him to be incarcerated again and to miss Christmas with his son anyway. But Carl was convinced that nothing else was more important than keeping this promise to his son. He was overlooking the promise he'd made to himself, to his family, and to the courts—the promise that he would complete his program and work on himself.

Part of working on himself was learning to communicate openly and honestly with his family members. This was something else he was neglecting to do as he continued making excuses why he "could not" tell his son that he would not be coming home for Christmas. Carl continued acting out, possibly as a way of self-sabotaging his recovery. He later admitted he hoped he would get thrown out of his program, then it could be the program's "fault" that he was unable to keep his promises to his son.

Carl was creating a lot of anxiety and stress in his life that all began from the so-called "trigger" of the upcoming holidays. Before that point, he had been very invested in his recovery; now, the emotions of holidays past, missed opportunities, euphoric recall for the "good ol' days," and lack of coping skills in early recovery were becoming evident in his struggle to move forward. After several prompted and uncomfortable phone calls and visits with his family and probation officer, Carl was able to accept that he was better off in treatment than he would have been if he'd left. He had to let go of his pride and ego and allow his son to experience his own disappointment. Carl was slowly able to get back on track and put things into perspective. He completed his program much later, as he learned he had so much more to work on.

One of the things he identified as being problematic for

him moving forward was the way holidays made him feel. He had made it through the first holidays of the year by being in a protected environment. Carl realized that if he felt this way now, once he left the security of his program, he would have to remain vigilant during the holidays in order to protect his serenity and sobriety.

Unfortunately, Carl was unable to embrace a crucial part of sobriety: acceptance. Shortly after he left, he relapsed. He continued to hold reservations about the things he could not accept, such as going to meetings to secure his sobriety, being honest in his communication with his family, and letting go of old people, places, and things. In essence, he carried his old baggage into a new year. The event of the holidays was a warning sign for Carl about how much more he needed to work on. This can be described as "the relapse before the relapse," a return to old behaviors and ways of dealing with conflict, anxiety, or difficult moments. The holidays have a way of bringing these things to the forefront.

Of course, individuals in recovery *can* learn to maneuver through these days and build a stronger foundation.

If you allow yourself to recognize how you are feeling, along with how are you coping, you will be armed with the tools necessary to avoid a risk of relapse during the holidays, and every day, as you grow stronger in your recovery.

For Reflection

- Think about holidays throughout the year. What are you looking forward to about them, and what do you anticipate might create anxiety for you?

- Are there any friends or family members who might create difficult interactions at a holiday celebration? If so, make a list of at least three things you can do to defuse the situation(s).

• What coping mechanisms are most helpful to you when you need to get through a bad day or a stressful event?

_____

_____

_____

_____

_____

_____

_____

_____

• Is there any holiday or special event that feels especially daunting to you? What emotions does that day bring up for you? How might you better manage those emotions?

_____

_____

_____

_____

_____

_____

_____

_____

- Does anything about Carl's story feel relatable to you? Have you faced similar difficult truths in your life? When that happened, how did you move forward?

_____

_____

_____

_____

_____

_____

_____

_____

CHAPTER EIGHT

Connecting to Your Passion

Have you ever asked children what they want to be when they grow up? One day, it might be a race-car driver. The next day, maybe an astronaut. They're ready each day to jump in and try new things without worrying about success or failure. Their enthusiasm is driven only by the question: "What makes me happy?"

Children do not limit themselves in the number of dreams they are passionate about. They live in the moment, carefree and exploring new ideas that might change from sunrise to sunset. But somewhere along the line as they grow older, they develop hesitation—maybe even fear—that stops them from pursuing their new ideas with the same conviction. Why does this happen? Is this just the normal transition from childhood to adulthood? And if so, why?

Why do we let go of our dreams and ideas as adults and become content with complacency? What does this do to the human spirit?

This chapter will explore the importance of finding a passion in life. Passion is particularly important for individuals in recovery. During active use and often in early recovery, individuals often state, "I loved getting high." It became part of their daily routine, not only as a physical need but also as a way of life. As a result, some people truly believe that their "passion" is getting high. If it were not for the pesky side effects such as health problems, risk of dying, financial struggles, legal woes, broken relationships, and so on, one might actually convince himself that using is a wonderful life. But the reality is no child ever says, "I want to be an addict when I grow up." Somewhere along the line, the child loses his vision and passion, replacing it with a false sense of happiness. This quickly becomes routine, which is followed by complacency and the lack of drive to change. Childhood dreams fall to the wayside, and the ability to create adult visions of a brighter future becomes compromised by addiction.

Recovery is an opportunity to recover one's passions. Although they might have changed drastically since childhood, dreams and goals can now manifest if they're pursued with the same enthusiasm and drive that were put into active drug use. This might have you scratching your head and saying, "What? You want me to pursue my dreams the way I did my addiction?" Absolutely! Think about it. When you were actively using, you probably did everything you could think of to make sure you had access to your drink or drug each day. You made time for it in your schedule, you made sure you had money for it—it might have been the first thing you thought of each day and the last thing you planned on before day's end. In other words, you made your addiction your priority.

Now, in sobriety, you have the opportunity to invest in your passions as much as you invested in your destruction. It is not only possible, it is also necessary. You must replace old habits with new, healthier ones in order to maintain long-term sobriety. Most people who are enjoying an extended period of sobriety have something in common: their continual pursuit of happiness. Notice the phrase is the "*pursuit* of happiness." Everyone has the right to pursue their dreams and figure out what makes them happy. For some it is money, fame, family, or friends. Others find their happiness in creating art or enjoying nature. Regardless of the dream, the pursuit is the real goal. Pursuing your passions should be an ongoing process throughout your life.

Keep an Open Mind

Many individuals in early sobriety overthink the concept of pursuing their passion. They believe it must be something life-altering or huge, but that is not true. In early recovery, many people are still trying to figure out who they are outside of the destructive relationship they had with drugs and alcohol. In active addiction, people often align themselves with other individuals who are self-destructing. This, of course, does not foster healthy discussions about dreams and goals; instead, it fosters negativity and avoidance and certainly subdues plans or dreams for the future.

Once you are on the road to recovery, you have an opportunity to try new things with new people and to re-evaluate previous experiences. For example, maybe you never liked fishing in the past. Or, maybe you just didn't like fishing with the people you were with at that time. Maybe you associate fishing with getting drunk or high, and the idea of fishing without substances no longer holds your interest. Or, maybe you just truly don't like fishing. Regardless, fishing is not really the issue at hand. What's important is the *pursuit* of finding out if there is more to the fishing experience than you'd considered in the past.

Keeping an open mind about new experiences can actually become your passion in early recovery. Pursuing new ideas, setting new goals, and fully exploring possibilities that you neglected when you were actively using is how you will continue to grow in your recovery. Limitations are set by fear. To live a life of addiction is to concede to these fears. As noted earlier in this chapter, as we grow older, we begin putting limitations on our ideas and dreams. We might say things like, "I missed my chance," or, "I'm too old to start something new now." This is giving in to the fears associated with change. It is the same thought process that keeps people in active use. You probably can relate to this if you felt like you were "too far gone" or "did not know where to start to change." If you're reading this now, though, you either got over that fear and took important steps to change your life or you are considering whether it is possible now—and of course it is! You're already doing something different. You're reading and doing research into recovery. You're pursuing your happiness and finding that your passion might be recovery itself!

People who do not pursue their passions in life are filled with regrets or resentment. For a person in recovery, this can be very dangerous, as it might spark some "Poor me!" thinking that creates excuses to slip back into a destructive lifestyle. People who try to live a life in which they are not truly comfortable are going against their nature, and that creates much of the anxiety, guilt, and shame common in addiction. Let's take a moment to dig into this.

Consider a person who continues to diet, never truly feeling like she's lost enough weight. She might have a genetic predisposition to be a particular body type, but she is determined that she must be a size four and will diet at any cost to ensure she meets her goal. What is really happening to this person? She is becoming weak and sick. She is trying to reach an unrealistic goal, one of becoming something she is simply not meant to be. She is fighting her own true nature. It's the same with drug addiction. In active use, you are trying to be something you are not meant to be, and it makes you sick. You are going against your nature. You are not fully recognizing the hopes or dreams you had as a child. This is why connecting to your passions in recovery is key to truly living and not just existing. When you just exist, you open that flood gate of regret and resentment, and you might find yourself back in the same place you were trying to get out of.

Existing vs. Living

Finding your passion does not necessarily mean finding out what you want to do with the rest of your life. There is a saying, "If you earn a living doing something you love, you will never work a day in your life." This is certainly true for some, but we must consider the reality of earning a living. There might not be many job openings for someone who has a passion for crocheting or bird-watching. Some people are able to discover ways to earn their living doing something they love, but for many, finding something they love to do when the work day is over is key to their happiness and overall well-being.

The human spirit must be nurtured in a healthy way to avoid boredom and the temptation of finding unhealthy means of escape from a life that's going against one's nature. Call it passion or a hobby, however you want to label it, without this key piece to the human experience, one really does simply exist—not live. We don't have to guess what happens to individuals who feel they are just existing. They become complacent or bored and often turn to substance use or other unhealthy behaviors to escape their daily stressors and routines.

Escape, Relax, Reward

When moving forward in recovery, or in life in general, finding something that motivates you is the key to living a full, productive life. Exploring new adventures with new people in unfamiliar places can be the push you need to find where your true nature lies. When one goal ends, quickly create another one so you will always feel that excitement for life. Allowing yourself to become bored or complacent in recovery is a dangerous path.

Know that your passion can, and might, change from one moment to the next, especially when you are in the process of uncovering what it might be. Be careful that you do not become fixated on any one goal, as Jen does in the story that follows. She became frustrated and bored with life when she realized she was unable to fulfill the one dream she had from years ago.

It is also important to stay realistic within your goals. Make sure you are maintaining balance between taking care of your adult needs and nurturing your childlike hopes and dreams. Life can and should be challenging. If you're not challenged, then you're not changing, and continued change is a key to maintaining long-term sobriety.

But for some people, life's daily challenges become so stressful, they turn to drugs and alcohol to escape, relax, and reward. When you find yourself feeling that way, remember those words: Escape. Relax. Reward—ERR! Think about that acronym and scream it out loud while you shake your first in the air. It's okay to get a little bit mad! Once you get that negative energy out, move forward and make a plan. Explore new, healthy ways to *escape* from your stressors. Then, make time to *relax*. As a child, you played without worry, creating innovative ideas and plans. Now, as an adult, you must find a way to do the same without incorporating harmful substances or unhealthy habits. *Rewards* are the things we give ourselves when we work hard and achieve goals we have set. Now, instead of telling yourself that you deserve to take a break by using drugs or alcohol, tell yourself that you deserve a better life—one filled with possibilities.

The reward of a better life means the opportunity to explore new horizons with the same wonderment you held as a child. It's the chance to live and not just exist. And most importantly, it's the freedom to quit going against your nature by allowing yourself to grow healthier each day, surrounding yourself with positive influences and experiencing life with optimism. Finding your passion can be a continual process that's filled with excitement. It is not something to fear or dread. It might even be something you already are doing that allows you to feel balanced and serene.

One last thing to consider when seeking your passion is that you are doing this for yourself. It doesn't matter what other people feel or think about it, and it doesn't have to manifest into something huge. It does not have to make you rich or famous. All it is meant to do is bring you the joy of accomplishing something that creates an energy within you, increasing your self-esteem and helping you reach self-actualization through your own expression in life.

Jen came to treatment for the second time feeling broken. She could not understand why she was unable to get her life on track. During her first stay in treatment, she had dealt with many of the issues she felt had plagued her since childhood, especially the friction she had with her older sister who had coached her through high school sports, helping her become eligible for a college scholarship.

Her sister, although well-meaning, was very harsh in her directives for success. She often pushed Jen beyond the limits of a normal child athlete, putting her down and calling her names if she did not perform to the level her sister expected. This followed Jen into her young-adult years in college, where she found herself competing at a more intense level. Jen was approached by a basketball scout who offered her a semi-pro position. This was a once-in-a-lifetime opportunity that could have helped her realize her dream of becoming a pro basketball player. But Jen began feeling pressured by the competition and by her sister, so she began using cocaine to enhance her stamina during practices. Eventually she began using steroids and other performance-enhancing drugs, as well. All the while, Jen's sister continued to push her to do more and be better. One day, during an important game, Jen suffered a devastating injury to her knee. She was hospitalized and needed surgery. She was crushed by this; her dreams and her career were put on hold. Jen had a passion for basketball and could not imagine herself doing anything other than playing on a pro team one day.

While in the hospital and throughout the recovery process from her injury, Jen received pain pills. As her addiction grew, her dreams of making it to the pro level diminished. She took a job in a very lucrative field, yet she was miserable. She was not living; she was simply existing. Eventually, her drug use graduated to heroin. Jen had lost all hope.

Jen was struggling, and she was scared. Back in treatment, she asked herself, *What can I do this time that will be any different?* She was worried that treatment "would not stick." After several weeks of dragging her feet through the process, Jen began digging deep and working hard to identify exactly what was missing in her life that caused her to relapse time after time. Everything always seemed to go back to her "glory days" when she was the star athlete. Yes, she had issues with her sister and her marriage was dysfunctional, but something about giving up on her dreams kept weighing on her mind, as well.

Her stress grew as Jen realized she was chasing a dream that could never really manifest now. She was older, her health had been compromised by years of drug use, and she had felony convictions due to the lifestyle that accompanied her use. So, that was it, she thought. She had missed her opportunity and was doomed to a life of drug use and broken dreams.

Her story could have ended there. But Jen fought back with the same spirit that had created a star athlete. Jen refused to concede to a life of complacency. She worked closely with her counselor to identify other areas of interest that might give her the spark that playing sports had. She continued working on repairing important relationships in her life, but this time she recognized that the most important relationship she had to work on was the one with herself. She began to dream again, and this time her dreams were grounded in reality. She accepted her limitations and created other goals for herself that were attainable.

After leaving treatment, Jen returned to working in the same lucrative field she had worked in before. She advanced in her company, taking exotic trips and living comfortably. All the while, she held on to her passion and love for sports. She became a volunteer coach for a girls' basketball team. Every weekend, she was in the gym doing what she loved and giving back to her community. Her relationship with her sister improved as she grew stronger in her recovery, gaining self-esteem and enjoying her life. Jen divorced her husband as she learned that putting herself first meant making tough decisions to let go of people who did not support the same dreams and goals she had.

Jen was able to pursue her happiness through another avenue besides alcohol and drugs. She recognized that there were many goals and dreams she could achieve in her lifetime, instead of just fixating on the one thing she could *not* do. She put the same effort into living as she had put into dying.

FOR REFLECTION

- What is one thing you would try or explore if you knew there was no fear of failing?

_____

_____

_____

_____

_____

_____

_____

_____

- What do you consider your passions in life? How do you nurture each of those passions?

_____

_____

_____

_____

_____

_____

_____

_____

_____

- Identify three new things you'd like to explore. These could be activities you'd like to try or topics you'd like to learn more about. Don't worry about time, money, or other constraints—just let yourself dream.

_____

_____

_____

_____

_____

_____

_____

_____

- What was one of your childhood dreams or goals? Did you accomplish it? Could it still be relevant to you today as an adult?

_____

_____

_____

_____

_____

_____

_____

_____

- What are some healthy tactics you've learned for escaping, relaxing, and rewarding yourself?

_____

_____

_____

_____

_____

_____

_____

_____

CHAPTER NINE

Medical Care and the Importance of Healthy Thinking

Every day, healthcare professionals see the connection between the mind and the body, as well as the effects that mental attitudes have on physical health.

One physician even recently noted that seventy percent of the people in his waiting room were there due to issues directly related to stress—everything from high blood pressure and migraines to irritable bowel syndrome. He then added that most people won't listen to him in that regard; they don't believe in the connection between the mind and the body.

Why is that?

It could be that most people would prefer a quick fix. Changing attitudes and using coping tools to manage life's inconveniences and lower stress levels is hard work, and it doesn't happen overnight. It can take weeks, months, or even years, depending on how long those previous attitudes have been ingrained.

But the connection between the mind and the body is clear, and in recovery, healthy thinking is a crucial component of healthy living.

Research supports the idea that our minds are powerful and can have a direct effect on our physical health. *Make yourself mind yourself.* In other words, be mindful of what you let come into your life. Filtering out the lies we tell ourselves can be a challenge, but those lies foster negativity, which affects our mood and attitude and causes decreased energy, motivation, and focus.

Much of our physical and emotional pain are about perception and how we deal with the influences around us. Grumbling and complaining don't alter the degree of our discomfort. They just promote self-pity, which can lead to feelings of depression and apathy. That, in turn, can lead to more discomfort, which leads to more self-pity, which leads to more discomfort, and so on.

It's a vicious cycle that starts in the mind.

Caring for and managing a client's emotional and mental health are just as vital to the process of addiction treatment as addressing the client's physical and medical needs. All four elements require an education process that takes time and patient instruction; in many cases, the client is being asked to overhaul his entire belief system, which is no easy task. That process begins with accurate and emphatic assessment.

Asking the Right Questions

When a client enters treatment at Adams Recovery Center, he is subject to an initial nursing assessment that helps the medical team settle on a course of treatment. However, this assessment only scratches the surface of what the individual might need in terms of care. In any treatment environment, ongoing day-to-day assessments are essential in determining how well a client is retaining and actively applying the information being taught.

The goal of any treatment program is for clients to successfully graduate, yes, but even more importantly, the goal is to give clients the tools and resources necessary to stay sober once they've left. Out in the real world, clients won't have someone there to hold their hands. They will have to use their own assessment skills and make decisions on their own.

They will need to be able to answer questions such as:

- Am I advocating for my own health care?
- Am I accurately assessing my pain? Or am I catastrophizing my symptoms?
- If I am exaggerating these symptoms, am I seeking immediate relief?
- Have I assessed how seeking immediate relief might jeopardize my sobriety?
- How receptive am I to instruction, guidance, and education?
- Overall, what is my level of receptivity?

Physicians, researchers, and mental-health professionals are continuing to assess the relationship between physical health and emotional stability.

As stated in the article "Forgiveness: Your Health Depends on It," by John Hopkins Medicine: "Conflict doesn't just weigh down the spirit; it can lead to physical health issues."[1]

Studies have found that the act of forgiveness can yield huge health benefits by lowering the risk of heart attack; improving cholesterol levels and sleep; and reducing pain, blood pressure, anxiety, depression, and stress.

This is significant in addiction treatment because all clients have spent at least part of their lives numbing their feelings and dulling their reactions. They don't completely understand how the body functions or how moods and emotions affect their physical being.

Putting aside the drugs or alcohol is just one piece of the puzzle. The client also must get in touch with his feelings and learn how to implement the proper tools to manage those feelings on a daily basis in order to maintain overall wellness—which, of course, includes sobriety.

Part of that maintenance is a daily assessment of how he feels, as well as determining the cause of those feelings. For someone recovering from addiction, this can be harder than it sounds. The world around him looks and feels completely different from what he's used to. He has to learn to look at the world through different eyes and use the skills he's learned in treatment to make different choices than the ones that led him into addiction in the first place.

---

1. Johns Hopkins Medicine. "Forgiveness: Your Health Depends on It," HopkinsMedicine.org, accessed February 6, 2018.

This includes changing how he perceives daily annoyances and health discomforts such as headaches and nausea. The tools he's gained in treatment help him learn how to stay healthy and manage stress without relying solely on over-the-counter (OTC) medications or other substances.

OTC MEDICATIONS

OTC medications are a major point of confusion for clients who don't understand the potential dangers of such medicines. To many people, using the word "danger" in relation to common medications can seem crazy. Unfortunately, it's not.

For those struggling with sobriety, OTC medications can become a new sort of crutch, a single step down the slippery slope back into addiction. A key tenet of sobriety is living life on life's terms, and OTC medications can become a way for someone to numb the pain, whether physical or emotional.

A client might say, "But heroin is my problem. Something that I can buy at the drugstore without a prescription is harmless, right?"

The truth is that relying on OTC medications can leave a person susceptible to falling back into old, unhealthy thought patterns, which can then lead back into the same unhealthy behaviors.

Sure, the OTC medications might work for a time, but eventually they can lose their effectiveness, failing to solve the perceived problem and leading the client to become desperate for something stronger, such as Percocet or Vicodin. From there, the road back to active addiction can be surprisingly short.

One point of emphasis with clients in treatment is the need to hydrate properly. Obviously, water is not the solution to every health issue, but many, if not most, clients suffer from dehydration due to drug use and overall lifestyle in active addiction. When they enter treatment, they're shocked to find out that proper hydration can "cure" a headache and improve their digestive health—no medication required.

Restoring Physical Health

Another key component of addiction treatment is rebuilding a client's physical health. Often, that starts with tearing down old belief systems about what is considered normal and natural.

One of the most pervasive and erroneous beliefs among clients is: *I shouldn't have pain.* There is a feeling of entitlement to comfort, the idea that pain is a bad thing that should be removed immediately. This belief leads to seeking instant gratification, which can sabotage recovery.

It takes time to educate patients that pain can actually have value. Pain lets us know that there is a larger problem somewhere within our bodies, something for which we need to find a real solution. Treating a symptom is not the same as treating the cause.

Masking the pain doesn't move us forward. It keeps us stuck, trapped in a vicious cycle: Once the mask has been removed, the pain returns, leading to searching for another way to mask the pain, only for it to come back again when *that* mask disappears.

A common obstacle is that clients often struggle to heed advice from medical personnel. They are used to self-medicating and serving as their own physicians. They believe that no one knows their needs as well as they do. They've believed for so long that their drug of choice is the only thing that makes them feel better, they can't see how much stress their addiction is actually causing them.

Lying, hiding, stealing, doing anything it takes obtain their next high—it's an exhausting lifestyle.

As clients work through treatment, they're amazed by the various symptoms they've experienced that were caused by stress. The book *The Mind-Gut Connection* states: "...an overactive fight-or-flight system with constantly elevated stress hormones circulating through our bodies can lead to serious mental illness, including anxiety disorders, panic disorders and depression. It can also cause a nasty assortment of stress-sensitive physical disorders, including obesity, metabolic syndrome, heart attacks, and strokes. And finally, the hyper-responsiveness of the brain-gut axis associated with this programing can cause chronic gut disorders like irritable bowel syndrome and chronic abdominal pain."[2]

---

2. Mayer, Emran. *The Mind-Gut Connection: How the Hidden Conversation within Our Bodies Impacts Our Mood, Our Choices, and Our Overall Health.* New York: Harper Wave, 2016.

Of course, recovery is inherently stressful as well, so a successful treatment program will take that into account and teach clients how to manage stress and understand its underlying causes. For example, if a client suffers from anxiety, it is important to determine whether that anxiety led to the drug use or if the drug use caused the anxiety.

Clients can learn any number of techniques to help quiet their anxiety. For some, deep breathing combined with guided, progressive muscle relaxation can be effective. For other clients, it's exercise and proper diet. In many cases, clients feel renewed energy and vitality simply from the structure of three meals a day and regular sleep patterns.

CREATING HEALTHY HABITS

Healthy habits enable clients to connect to their own moods and emotions, as well as with the world around them. Staying connected to medical support is also a critical piece of recovery. No two cases are the same. Some clients need mental-health medications, while others need referrals to specialists for acute medical conditions. Continuity of care helps individuals understand the mind-body connections that comprise good health, and that understanding allows them to take responsibility for caring for themselves.

In their previous lifestyle, the only connection they understood was how to get their drug of choice. In treatment, they learn to access their real needs—both physical and emotional—and learn to identify new ways of coping.

They can take ownership over their attitudes and mind-sets because they've gained confidence through education.

They've learned how to manage stress-related events, how diet might cause mood fluctuations, and how sleep affects the body. Being able to care for oneself, to advocate for oneself, gives a client a renewed sense of purpose.

For clinicians, it's immensely gratifying to hear a client say, "I never thought I would feel so good. My skin is clearer. My doctor says my blood pressure is down and my sugar is better." It's edifying to see them deal with headaches and colds by moderating their sugar intake and managing their stress levels.

Of course, restoring health is a process, a methodical chipping away at old patterns, beliefs, and behaviors. Clients often will take one step forward and two steps back as they learn to see all of the options before them. It takes time and patience to realize that quitting at sobriety is not one of them.

As clients put one foot in front of the other on the most difficult days, they begin to develop a "new" normal. They learn to feel rather than to fear, to cope rather than to become anxious. They form new habits and begin to respect themselves and those who help in their care. They come to appreciate and celebrate their achievements, such as learning to effectively communicate their needs to get appropriate care. They learn to trust themselves and the medical professionals who can help them.

Most importantly, they learn that the control they thought they had in their addiction was simply a lie and that true control comes through focusing their energy into implementing strategies that support a healthier lifestyle.

Addiction might start in the mind, but so does recovery.

• • • WENDY AND ELENA'S STORIES • • •

Wendy, a client in her thirties, was shocked to discover some of the changes that slowly but surely took place as she moved through treatment and recovery and into sobriety. She was amazed to discover how effective something as simple and often overlooked as drinking water can be.

She said, "I can't believe how different I feel drinking water. I have more energy, and it is amazing. Honestly, I didn't believe it. Seriously, I thought, *What could drinking more water do*? But now it makes sense, because the more I see how I didn't take care of myself out there, didn't eat right or care about drinking water, the more my body really suffered."

Elena, a client in her late forties, shared how drinking more water had led to a different experience: natural and healthy weight loss.

"My doctors couldn't believe how good I looked when I went for a visit, from my skin color to how much weight I had lost," she reported. "I feel great, and I have to tell you this weight thing is a big deal for me. More often than not, it's what has caused me to relapse in the past. I feel so good from finding out some basic, simple things that I can do to feel healthy about myself and my lifestyle."

For Reflection

- Consider your reaction to physical pain. Is your first response to reach for a pill, or do you know other strategies for feeling better?

_____

_____

_____

_____

_____

_____

_____

_____

- What do you think about the concept that over-the-counter medications can be a gateway to using harder substances and falling into active addiction?

_____

_____

_____

_____

_____

_____

_____

_____

- How is your relationship with medical providers? Do you have a doctor or therapist you can confide in? Do you struggle with trusting others to help you feel better?

_____

_____

_____

_____

_____

_____

_____

_____

- What have you observed about your own body-mind connection? How do your emotions affect your physical health? How do exercise and proper diet affect your mental well-being?

_____

_____

_____

_____

_____

_____

_____

_____

_____

- Think of a time when you advocated for yourself and clearly communicated your needs. How did you feel? What was the outcome?

  _____

  _____

  _____

  _____

  _____

  _____

  _____

  _____

CHAPTER TEN

Aftercare Options

One of the biggest questions we hear at Adams Recovery Center is, "What should be the next step after someone graduates from treatment?" Our answer is simple: It's complicated.

That's why we start this chapter with a story, to illustrate the importance of thinking through the various aftercare avenues and what is appropriate for each individual case.

••• CLAUDETTE'S STORY •••

Claudette had just completed a six-month residential treatment and had been informed by her counselor that, per American Society of Addiction Medicine (ASAM) criteria, she qualified for intensive outpatient services (IOP). It was recommended that Claudette live in a sober-living accommodation and attend IOP. Claudette agreed but then reported that she was going to go back home for a few days to get some things settled.

She was encouraged by her peers and her counselor not to go because her mother was addicted to cocaine and had come into money through an inheritance. Claudette said that a few days at home would not affect her sobriety and that if she couldn't be at her mom's house for a few days and not use, then she'd never be able to make it anyway. Claudette went back to her mother's house and passed away just a few days later from an apparent overdose.

MAKING THE CHOICE

It's hard not to wonder if Claudette would still be alive if she had taken the recommendation of her counselor. But we don't order clients to do anything—the choice is entirely theirs. Here's what's behind the suggestions we make.

For some people, we highly recommend IOP. For others, we will recommend outpatient services, and for others we will suggest sober-living accommodations tied to sober recovery groups. Every person has unique needs that must be met in order to maintain sobriety.

In Ohio, IOP is defined as attending nine hours and one minute of group counseling each week. Typically, that will be spread over three days per week for about three hours per session. Regular outpatient treatment can range from nine hours or fewer depending on the individual case. At our agency, this typically consists of a two-hour group session each week and an hour of individual counseling.

We believe that anyone who is leaving treatment will benefit from continued structure and support. We also evaluate based on standard ASAM criteria. Using these criteria, we will evaluate an individual's emotional needs, withdrawal risk, medical conditions, readiness for change, relapse potential, and recovery environment before recommending the appropriate level of care.

There is no one size that fits all in aftercare. For some people, continuing to attend group counseling might seem exhausting after they have just completed six months of groups every day. For others, attending groups three days a week is exactly the accountability and therapy they need. We've also found that certain people do very well with individual counseling because they need to talk to someone about their issues but don't need peer feedback.

Peer-support meetings (Alcoholics Anonymous, Narcotics Anonymous, Smart Recovery, Celebrate Recovery, etc.) have existed for years and have shown success, as well. Again, it depends on the individual. Many people who attend sober-support meetings and/or live in a sober-living environment find that is just the right mix to maintain their sobriety. They benefit from getting support in their meetings and having accountability at home.

Some individuals do not want to go to sober living due to their family obligations. That's entirely understandable. That said, we encourage clients to look at what is best for their long-term sobriety, because going back into the same old environment can lead to using again. Furthermore, if an individual has just completed a three- to six-month rehabilitation program, it might feel overwhelming to return to an environment that isn't as structured as treatment.

In every case, clients must weigh the pros and cons for themselves. At our agency, we emphasize two primary considerations: getting that ASAM assessment to determine what level of care is most appropriate, and remembering the importance of placing yourself and your sobriety first.

CHAPTER ELEVEN

Frequently Asked Questions

Can't I or my loved one just stop using? What's the big deal?
Unfortunately, that's not how it works. By the time an addiction becomes an addiction, there is a reliance upon the substance. To put it simply, the person's brain has been "rewired" by the substance, and work needs to be done to set it straight. Obviously, this is much more complicated than this brief answer, and we encourage you to read through this book to get a better grasp on addiction and its components. In the meantime, though, start eradicating that belief that the solution is telling someone, "Just stop it!" Although there are some people out there who have been able to "just stop it," that is not the reality for most.

Okay, so I need help. What type of treatment do I need? Do I really need to go to "rehab"?
Yay! Recognizing the need for help is a wonderful first step! The type of treatment you need is dependent upon a lot of factors, though. The best way to determine which type of treatment might be appropriate for you is to seek out a clinician or a social services agency and have an assessment done. They then can recommend options to you and

connect you to resources. And yes, you might need to go to "rehab" (we prefer "residential treatment"), and that's okay. A huge mistake many people make is not pursuing the best treatment option(s) for them because it's a big change and it's scary. Don't hold yourself back. Take the leap!

Why do I have to follow some type of program? Isn't my addiction unique to me?

Sort of. The reasons you use, specific issues that contributed to or resulted from your use, and the way you process things are unique to you, yes. But addiction itself is pretty cut and dried: a reliance upon a substance or substances. There are various ways to approach treating addiction, but again, even those are pretty similar: promote abstinence from substances, address issues related to use, and then make positive changes to support sobriety. If you find yourself thinking your addiction is so different and unique that there isn't a treatment option out there for you, then honestly, you might be using that as an excuse to continue using.

Will my brain ever go back to "normal"?

Yes and no. Here's the obvious part: Drugs and alcohol have a major impact on the brain and its functions. The unknown parts are exactly how and to what extent drugs and alcohol have affected *your* brain. That depends in part on the types or combinations of substances you used. Research provides a promising outlook, though, and overall it suggests that those who maintain long-term abstinence from substances see improvement (and usually a complete return) of their brain functions.

Will the cravings and urges ever go away?

Maybe. Again, it all depends on the person. Cravings and urges are a totally normal thing, and it's also totally normal to have them on occasion even after weeks, months, or years of sobriety. As we said, the brain is changed by addiction. After years of dependence on a substance, the brain isn't going to let go that easily. It will take time for cravings to go away, but they will eventually. As you take steps away from using and learn new coping skills, the urges and cravings will lessen. When they do occur, try to see it as an opportunity to learn how to cope with them in a healthy way. Rather than see it as a weakness or a sign that you aren't "getting better," see it as your brain healing and as part of pursuing a better life.

I keep hearing about "ninety meetings in ninety days." Do I have to do that?

A lot of clients ask us this question, and we usually don't give a direct reply because we want people to explore their own options. We bring in several types of support groups at our treatment centers so people can explore which ones, if any, might be helpful for them post-treatment. If you want to pursue a ninety-in-ninety because you believe it will be beneficial to your sobriety, then great! Try it out! Here's the thing, though: You also need to be realistic. Do you have the ability to accomplish this goal? If life happens one day and prevents you from making it to a meeting, will that cause you major distress? The issue that sometimes occurs with ninety-in-ninety is that all-or-nothing thinking creeps in. People will miss a meeting and feel ashamed or like they failed rather than recognizing the reality of the situation: Life happens, mistakes happen, and ninety-in-ninety is a choice, not a requirement, for sobriety.

Is it okay to be in a relationship early in recovery?

This is a two-part answer. The first part is for those who are already in a relationship. If you are in a relationship while in active addiction, a lot of work probably will need to be done when entering into sobriety. Whether both of you were in addiction or not, addiction brings toxicity into relationships that will need to be addressed. This might mean improving communication, ceasing enabling, addressing a lack of trust, and so on. Really look at the relationship and your feelings toward it. Also, don't fall into the trap of staying together just to stay together. If it's not working, forcing it will just make things more toxic.

For those of you who are single and looking to mingle, here's our take on it: We are not going to throw out a timeline of when you can be in a relationship. What we can say, though, is that you might want to ask yourself some questions. What are your intentions for entering into a relationship? Are you currently supporting yourself both emotionally and financially? Are you able to deal with conflict in healthy ways? Do you have goals? Will entering into a relationship jeopardize any of those goals? What we tend to see in early recovery is that people enter into relationships quickly because it allows them to focus on someone besides themselves. It also satisfies the codependency that often comes with addiction. So be honest with yourself. And if you can't do that, maybe a relationship isn't the best choice right now.

Can I still hang around my old friends?

We get this question a lot, and it baffles us. We know it's difficult to accept, but hanging around old friends with whom you used to use is probably one of the worst decisions you can make. Hanging out with people who are still in active addiction will only keep you in that lifestyle. Even if you don't directly use, you're surrounding yourself with what you are trying to get away from.

Okay, so what if they got sober as well? That might be okay, but we've seen many people have issues with this, especially if the thought patterns and behaviors associated with using are still present. Many times, people forget about the reality of the past and focus on "the good ol' days" when hanging out with old using friends, and it can lead to some dangerous thoughts and/or actions. Be selective about the people with whom you surround yourself. Don't hang out with old "friends" just because it's comfortable and easy. Unfortunately, pursuing a sober life is not always comfortable and easy, but it is worth it. The relationships you form in sobriety will be much more meaningful and supportive than any based on substance use.

My loved one is in early recovery. How can I best support him?

First things first: Listen to the person. *Really* listen, without any preconceived notions or beliefs. Let your loved one communicate with you about his thoughts and feelings without judgment. Utilize empathy and understanding to bridge connections. This might be hard, because you might not entirely understand where he is coming from. You might even have difficulty grasping the concept of addiction, and that's okay. Seeking to better understand is a great step in supporting someone. Maybe even ask how you can support your loved one, how you can help when he is struggling. The truth is, your loved one will struggle, and having a solid and nonjudgmental support system is a wonderful asset in sobriety.

Now, we want to make it clear that we don't associate "support" with "money." We are talking about emotional support here. Your monetary support is entirely up to you, and we encourage you to set boundaries with it.

That leads us to this advice: Take care of yourself! Addiction is not a single-person issue; it extends outward. Your loved one living with addiction probably had a huge effect on you. Looking at your own issues and the stresses that arose during that time will be very helpful for you. Seeking out counseling and support groups for families and significant others of addicts could be a great step, in addition to possibly seeking out individual counseling. Addressing your own issues so you and your loved one can grow together is another great way to be supportive.

Websites

SAMHSA.gov—The Substance Abuse and Mental Health Services Administration has educational materials on addiction and mental health.

CDC.gov—The Centers for Disease Control and Prevention website offers statistics and other helpful medical information about alcohol and drug abuse.

DrugAbuse.gov—The National Institute on Drug Abuse provides research-based facts and information about addiction.

NAMI.org—The National Alliance on Mental Illness website includes information and resources for seeking help and support.

AA.org—The Alcoholics Anonymous website provides information about AA and how to find meetings in your area.

NA.org—The Narcotics Anonymous website provides information about NA and how to find meetings in your area.

Al-anon.alateen.org—Al-Anon provides support for family members and loved ones of problem drinkers.

Nar-anon.org—Nar-Anon provides support for family members and loved ones of those struggling with addiction.

SmartRecovery.org—The website provides information about SMART Recovery and how to find meetings in your area.

CelebrateRecovery.com—The website provides information about Celebrate Recovery, which is a Christ-centered program, and how to find meetings in your area.

Books and articles

American Psychiatric Association. *Diagnostic and Statistical Manual of Mental Disorders (5th Edition).* Washington, D.C.: American Psychiatric Publishing, 2013.

Blanco, C., Okuda, M., Wang, S., Liu, S., and Olfson, M. (2014). "Testing the Drug Substitution Switching-Addictions Hypothesis." *JAMA Psychiatry,* 71(11), 1246. doi:10.1001/jamapsychiatry.2014.1206

Foote, Jeffrey, Carrie Wilkens, Nicole Kosanke, and Stephanie Higgs. *Beyond Addiction: How Science and Kindness Help People Change.* New York: Scribner, 2014.

Frankl, Viktor. *Man's Search for Meaning.* Boston: Beacon Press, 2006.

Glasner-Edwards, Suzette. *The Addiction Recovery Skills Workbook: Changing Addictive Behaviors Using CBT, Mindfulness, and Motivational Interviewing Techniques.* Oakland, Calif.: New Harbinger Publications, 2016.

James, John W. and Russell, Friedman. *The Grief Recovery Handbook: 20th Anniversary Edition.* N.p.: HarperCollins, 2009.

Kübler-Ross, Elisabeth. *On Death and Dying: What the Dying Have to Teach Doctors, Nurses, Clergy and Their Own Families*. London: Routledge, 2009.

Sheff, David. *Beautiful Boy: A Father's Journey Through His Son's Addiction*. New York: Mariner, 2008.

Spiegelman, Erica. *Rewired: A Bold New Approach to Addiction and Recovery*. Hobart, New York: Hatherleigh Press, 2015.

Williams, Rebecca E., and Julie S. Kraft. *The Mindfulness Workbook for Addiction: A Guide to Coping with the Grief, Stress, and Anger that Trigger Addictive Behaviors*. Oakland, Calif.: New Harbinger Publications, 2012.

Additional books by KiCam Projects

Adams Recovery Center. *Accept, Reflect, Commit: Your First Steps to Addiction Recovery*. Georgetown, Ohio: KiCam Projects, 2017.

Adams Recovery Center. *Addiction, Recovery, Change: A How-To Manual for Successfully Navigating Sobriety*. Georgetown, Ohio: KiCam Projects, 2016.

Leder, Sharon. *The Fix: A Father's Secrets, A Daughter's Search*. Georgetown, Ohio: KiCam Projects, 2017.

Thorngren, John T. *Salvation on Death Row: The Pamela Perillo Story*. Georgetown, Ohio: KiCam Projects, 2018.

Also available from KiCam Projects:

Addiction, Recovery, Change
A How-To Manual for Successfully Navigating Sobriety
by ADAMS RECOVERY CENTER

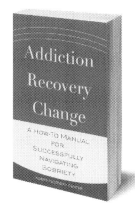

Whether you're building a new life or supporting a loved one, this is the resource you need to meet the everyday challenges of staying clean and sober.

$11.95 / 112 pages

Accept, Reflect, Commit
Your First Steps to Addiction Recovery
by ADAMS RECOVERY CENTER

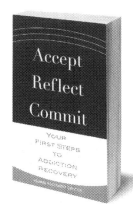

This practical guidebook prepares readers for the recovery journey, explaining what to expect along the way and how to choose the right treatment option..

$12.95 / 176 pages

Also available from KiCam Projects:

The Fix
A Father's Secrets,
A Daughter's Search
by SHARON LEDER

Through the eyes of Sara Katz,
author Sharon Leder makes peace
with her family's history as she
explores her childhood as the
daughter of a heroin addict who lost
his battle with drugs.

$19.95 / 256 pages

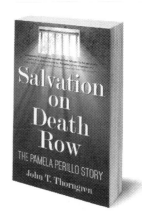

Salvation on Death Row
The Pamela Perillo Story
by JOHN T. THORNGREN

A life of abuse and addiction led
Pamela Perillo to Texas's Death
Row, where Pamela found new life
through sobriety and faith.

$19.95 / 224 pages

Available now on KiCamProjects.com and Amazon.com.

To learn more about Adams Recovery Center,
please visit AdamsRecoveryCenter.org,
call 513-575-0968,
or email info@adams-recovery-center.org.